MW01140697

# Massage

## *The Best Massage Techniques From Around The World*

By Ace McCloud
Copyright © 2016

# Disclaimer

The information provided in this book is designed to provide helpful information on the subjects discussed. This book is not meant to be used, nor should it be used, to diagnose or treat any medical condition. For diagnosis or treatment of any medical problem, consult your own physician. The publisher and author are not responsible for any specific health or allergy needs that may require medical supervision and are not liable for any damages or negative consequences from any treatment, action, application or preparation, to any person reading or following the information in this book. Any references included are provided for informational purposes only. Readers should be aware that any websites or links listed in this book may change.

# Table of Contents

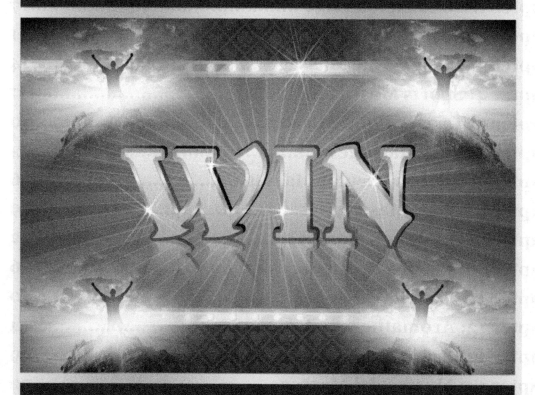

DEDICATED TO THOSE WHO ARE PLAYING THE GAME OF LIFE TO

KEEP ON PUSHING AND NEVER GIVE UP!

Ace McCloud

# Be sure to check out my website for all my Books and Audio books.

## www.AcesEbooks.com

# Introduction

I want to thank you and congratulate you for buying the book, "Massage: The Best Massage Techniques From Around the World."

This book contains proven steps and strategies on how to determine the best type of massage therapy for your needs. It will introduce you to the best massage techniques from around the globe, so come along with me and discover all the incredibly inventive massage techniques developed over the last thousand years and how you can utilize them to heal your body and make your life happier and healthier.

Massage therapy is a form of healing touch. It offers an excellent way to help your body relax, recover from stress, heal injuries, while having therapeutic effects on the mind, emotions and body. Massage therapy has been utilized for thousands of years to treat muscle tension, chronic pain, and a variety of physical, emotional, spiritual, and psychological issues.

During massage therapy, another person, usually a licensed massage therapist, discerns the parts of your body that need special attention and then applies pressure to those areas using fingers, hands, elbows, feet and special devices to relieve stress, release muscle tension, and reduce pain. The focus of the massage is mainly on your muscles, tissues, skin, and joints.

In this book, you will explore the mechanics of a wide range of massage therapies and how you can utilize them yourself to get much needed relief. You will be provided with plenty of information so you can decide whether Shiatsu, deep tissue, Swedish, trigger point, or another type of massage will best serve your needs. You will also learn about Thai massage, myofascial massage, reflexology, and massage that utilizes hot stones and aromatherapy. We will discuss sports-related massage and massage to facilitate a woman's pregnancy. We will even discuss – tastefully, of course – Erotic and Tantric massage, two massage forms that can be incredibly enjoyable.

Be prepared to discover all you need to know to bring your massage skills to the next level.

# Chapter 1: Swedish Massage

Swedish massage comes from, unsurprisingly, Sweden. This is probably what you are thinking of when you use the word "massage." Swedish massage relaxes the body by manipulating muscles in gliding strokes. It involves pressure and manipulation with the therapist's hands, palms, forearms and elbows in firm kneading motions, drum-like tapping, bending and stretching, or long smooth strokes.

## Benefits

The benefits of Swedish massage are many. Its primary accomplishment is to force oxygen into your bloodstream, improving your circulation. It also removes toxins by flushing them out of your muscles and persuades these muscles to release their tension while at the same time encouraging them to become more flexible. Swedish massage does not only affect your physical body, but also offers mental and emotional benefits. Stress is relieved, relaxation is achieved, and the mind is allowed to rest.

Muscles and joints tend to loosen under the hands of a Swedish massage practitioner and those nasty knots where your muscles bunch up will untangle and flow smoothly. Muscle spasms often cease and muscle tissues are reinvigorated. If you are prone to muscle cramps, particularly in the legs and calves, a Swedish massage can provide both treatment and preventative measures. By increasing your blood circulation, it also improves skin and muscle tone.

If you have an injury, Swedish massage can promote healing. It decreases pain, and can reduce the symptoms of arthritis, carpal tunnel, asthma, chronic fatigue, fibromyalgia, headaches, and TMJ, to name just a few. Swedish massage can also help with insomnia, depression and anxiety. It leaves the recipient with a feeling of well-being and may even improve one's concentration.

## Origins

Per Henrik Ling, fencing instructor at the University of Stockholm, developed this form of massage in the 1830s. He had injured his elbows and nothing else seemed to cure the problem, so he began to experiment. He started by tapping the elbow area with his fingers and using short drum-like strokes to stimulate the area around both elbows. Sure enough, his injury improved.

Swedish massage was introduced to the United States by brother physicians, Charles and George Taylor, in the 1850s. It took the country by storm. Today, Swedish massage is looked upon as a valid method for treating sore muscles and to enhance health and increase a person's general sense of well-being.

## How it Works

You've probably watched people receiving massages in the movies. Perhaps you have indulged in a massage at one time or another. In either case, you're already aware that Swedish massage is performed with the recipient in the nude, albeit tastefully covered with a sheet or towel. If it is particularly uncomfortable to receive treatment in the nude, most therapists will allow a client to keep their underwear on. The draping, which is removed from an area being massaged and then covered again, provides not only for a client's modesty, but also traps the body heat to keep the muscles relaxed and supple.

Oil is applied to the body as a lubricant, to facilitate the fluid, gliding motions of the therapist's hands on the skin. Frequently, the oil is tinged with a fragrant essence, to enhance relaxation.

A massage may last anywhere from 30 to 60 minutes. The movements and pressure applied by the therapist warm the skin and the muscles, breaking up any knots and adhesions and facilitating blood circulation.

The client initially lies face down on a massage table. The face is cradled in a horseshoe-shaped cushion that allows for uninhibited breathing. The massage usually starts by working the back, and then moves on to the legs. After the client turns face up, the therapist works the arms, the neck, and the top of the shoulders.

## Techniques

Specific techniques are unique to Swedish massage. Each one accomplishes a different purpose, but the overall objective is to move the toxins out of the muscles and facilitate their relaxation.

**Effleurage** is the most common technique. It consists of flowing and gliding motions on the skin that move toward the heart. The therapist may trace the contours of the body using hands and palms. Light and constant pressure is applied by the hands. The upper back, neck, shoulders, legs and arms benefit from effleurage.

**Petrissage** uses a kneading motion, as if working on bread dough. The therapist takes a handful of flesh and lifts, rolls, and squeezes it between hands and fingers to smooth out any knots or lumps in the muscles and facilitate the removal of toxins.

**Friction** is used to affect the deeper muscles. This is where the therapist uses body weight to press flat palms down onto the client. In different situations, the pads of the thumbs and fingers, the knuckles, or the backs of the forearms may be "pressed" into service to accomplish friction. With this technique, pressure starts light but increases steadily up to a point. It then is released gradually. Sliding or circular motions may be employed when applying friction.

**Vibration** is another technique that consists of the therapist gently shaking – or vibrating – the flesh with the hand or fingertips. It is a quick light motion that encourages muscles to loosen up and let go of toxins.

**Tapotiment** is a tapping or drum-like movement that is choppy and rhythmic. It stimulates the skin and muscles. Three basic actions are employed:

1. **Cupping** occurs when the hands form a cup shape, with the fingers folded under at the lower knuckles. The thumbs are held against the side of the palm. In this technique, the therapist strikes the flesh with cupped hand in rapid succession, alternating left and right palms.

2. **Hacking** is, well, hacking. It consists of a Karate chopping motion where the sides of the hands strike the skin, impacting the muscles beneath.

3. **Pummeling** uses the fists to gently nudge the buttocks and thigh muscles to relax and release their toxins.

Tapotiment may be too violent for some people, but many find it highly invigorating. As you might imagine, this technique can tire out both therapist and recipient. If implemented in excess, it can over-stimulate both muscles and nerves. As a result, tapotiment is usually performed toward the end of a massage, when the recipient is most relaxed and may be falling asleep. It serves as a not-too-rude awakening for the client.

## Equipment

Swedish Massage is performed on a table that places the client a little lower than the practitioner's waist. The face cushion is for the client's comfort; other cushions may be placed under the head or knees while the client is lying face up. Oils are a vital part of Swedish massage equipment. Most therapists employ vegetable-based oils, most often olive oil. These oils can be scented or not and may contain some vitamins. They do not clog the pores.

## Contraindications

Although there is no indication of problems caused by Swedish massage, there are several conditions under which it should be avoided. If you have a stomach or intestinal bug, cancel your appointment. If you have a recently broken bone, torn ligaments or damaged tendons, your massage therapist will avoid working those areas; the same goes if you have a bad sprain. Open wounds will not be massaged and if you have an inflamed area or a sizeable bruise, your massage therapist will avoid those regions of your body as well. Varicose veins will be avoided, as well as any area that has been through recent surgery.

Be very careful if you have a heart problem, suffer from high blood pressure, are fighting cancer, have a history of blood clots, or are taking a blood thinner. Your massage therapist will need to know about these conditions in order to treat you effectively and safely. If you have any of these conditions, you should restrict your massage treatments to only professionally trained therapists.

There isn't much bad that can happen with Swedish Massage, but there is always the chance of dislodging a blood clot. Most people do not have any problems except that they may feel a little sore after a session. Drinking a lot of water before and after can minimize or prevent the pain, but any pain should go away within a day or so.

Before your first massage with a specific therapist, you will probably have a consultation. This is the time to provide essential information that can inform your therapist's work with you. Any therapist will need to know your medical history, all medications you are taking and any injuries you have sustained. If you have any allergies, your consultation is the time to make them known. You don't want a relaxing massage to turn into an uncomfortable rash or a congested respiratory system.

You should tell the therapist your current physical trouble points. Point out any area of your body that is particularly painful. If you are pregnant, you should avoid Swedish massage unless the practitioner is trained in pregnancy massage. Also be sure to tell the therapist if you prefer a light or firm touch. Don't give up entirely if you're sick on the day of the massage; just reschedule your appointment for a later date if you are feeling under the weather.

# Chapter 2: Shiatsu Massage

Shiatsu massage was developed around 1320 in Japan by Akashi Ichi. Shiatsu is a Japanese word meaning finger pressure. The massage utilizes the fingers, thumbs, and palms to work on the skin and the underlying muscles. It employs the use of joint manipulation, movement and sometimes palpitation. This form of massage is performed on a fully clothed individual.

This form of massage focuses on the life energy that courses through our bodies. This energy is called Qi or Chi. Shiatsu works to free the body from energy blockages so that the Chi can flow freely throughout the body, infusing it with energy and health. The energy is stimulated and causes the body to feel calm and relaxed. When the energy can once again flow freely, it is believed that the body self-adjusts to a healthier condition.

## Benefits

While there are no scientific studies to document the benefits of Shiatsu massage, there are centuries of anecdotal evidence. It increases energy and relieves stress. Muscular pain is often removed entirely by letting the energy flow unimpeded through the body. While Shiatsu treats the physical body as a whole, it also has strong healing effects on mind, emotions and spirit. It is known to help digestive issues, migraines, skin problems, muscle aches, PMS, fatigue, insomnia, depression, and anxiety. Some people swear that if they participate in Shiatsu at least twice a month, it protects them from the effects of stress.

## How it Works

Shiatsu borrowed some of its philosophy from acupuncture, including the meridians defined by Chinese medicine. It was originally practiced in Japan but within the last century or so has become well known around the world.

During World War II, Shiatsu was banned in the United States, probably for no other reason than that Japan was the enemy. However, it was soon reinstated in America and now enjoys a respected place among other forms of massage. A Shiatsu college was formed In the 1940s, giving added credibility to this practice.

## Description
Shiatsu massage utilizes pressure that is applied to targeted areas of the body. Stimulation of these areas improves the flow of Qi (or Chi), the life force. Practitioners use their palms, fingers and thumbs to perform the massage. They apply pressure in rhythmic circles for about two to eight seconds and then gradually release the pressure. While the pressure is applied, certain points on the body may feel tender and uncomfortable, but most recipients describe this as "good" or healing pain.

A low table is commonly the surface on which the recipient lies. Often a futon is used; a mattress on the floor also works well.

The client is fully clothed throughout the massage. You may be asked to follow specific exercises for breathing or visualization. You may be asked to move in specific ways and hold yoga-like poses.

Before the practitioner even touches a client, the two will hold a consultation. Physical information is passed on as well as the recipient's mental and emotional state. The session may take 40 to 50 minutes and the recipient must rest for about one hour after the massage. Results may not be realized until a few days after a session, but in many cases, changes may be immediately apparent.

## Techniques

**Pressure** - The practitioner kneels on the floor and uses palms, fingers or thumbs to apply pressure using body weight. A low table or mattress on the floor is used to facilitate the therapist's leaning in to apply pressure. There are no quick movements In Shiatsu, everything is done slowly. The therapist's pressure increases slowly and is released slowly. Breathing and visualization exercises are utilized in order to aid in freeing the Qi to circulate. The practitioner moves their body to aid the Qi in flowing to where it is needed.

**Stretching** - Muscles store lactic acid, which must be released to avoid knots and muscle pain. Stretching frees toxins from the muscle fibers and releases trapped Qi. Stretches are accomplished slowly and the recipient only stretches as far as possible without causing discomfort.

**Kneading** the muscles improves circulation and helps to flush out toxins from muscles. The practitioner takes skin and muscle between thumb and fingers or grabs flesh with the hands and squeezes.

**Manipulation of Joints** - Joints are moved in the direction of normal motion. No pressure is applied during manipulation. The practitioner will manipulate a joint only as far as is comfortable for the recipient.

**Pounding** stimulates the skin on the surface to improve circulation. It is said that Qi resides close to the skin. The practitioner pounds a client with the hands. Their hands flop up and down in rhythmic motion. They may also use their fists or clasp their hands together perform the pounding action.

## Equipment

A low table or mattress on the floor is where Shiatsu takes place. Cushions are helpful to provide support behind the head or under the knees.

## Contraindications

Not everyone should pursue Shiatsu massage therapy. Pregnant women should be especially careful to only place themselves under the care of a practitioner who is trained in Shiatsu massage during pregnancy. Chemotherapy or radiation treatment patients should avoid it entirely, as should individuals with heart disease or thinned blood. Do not attend a massage session if you have inflammation of the skin, open wounds, massive bruises, tumors, recently fractured bones, or surgery of any kind. If you have an abdominal hernia, your therapist can be alerted to avoid massaging that area.

There should be no negative side effects from Shiatsu Massage. You may be a little sore for a day or two, if you are not used to it. Many people feel immediate pain relief with no side effects at all. At the same time, it is advisable to keep yourself well hydrated for a couple days after the massage, in order to facilitate the removal of toxins from the body.

## Logistics

Do not eat a heavy meal before heading out for a massage. Shiatsu is highly personal, so the techniques employed during a massage depend on the needs and preferences of the recipient. Most people receive a massage every two to three weeks. Many report that a regular maintenance program keeps their meridians open and the Qi flowing. If they notice blockage, they can always go back for an extra session. When the Qi flows freely, a client is less likely to become sick or despondent.

# Chapter 3: Deep Tissue Massage

Deep Tissue massage is somewhat similar to Swedish Massage but the pressure put on the body by the therapist is much greater. This type of massage is not recommended for anyone who has never before had a massage, simply because of the intensity of the experience. Even those experienced in Swedish or Shiatsu massage often report feeling some pain. The fear is that a newbie might be dissuaded from ever having a massage again if they start at this point!

Deep tissue massage more resembles a session of physical therapy than a relaxing massage. The client needs to put a little work into the massage, too. A deep tissue massage enables the deep layers within muscle tissue to become aligned and it also gives connective tissue more flexibility. The therapist works on muscle tissue, tendons and fascia that protect the joints, muscles and bones. Finger pressure is used in very slow, but extremely firm strokes on areas that have been treated with warm oil. This massage releases large amounts of toxins into the blood stream, so hydration, both before and after, is essential.

## Benefits

According to the University of Maryland Medical Center, deep tissue massage is very effective in a variety of ways. It greatly increases blood flow and circulation and can help with inflammation and muscle tension. It is often used to break down scar tissue by increasing lymphatic circulation and thus resulting in greater flexibility.

This massage is good for rehabbing from injuries, and for treating pain, osteoarthritis, tennis elbow, fibromyalgia, chronic fatigue, sciatica, and muscle spasms. It often helps increase range of motion that has been restricted by injury or stiffness. It helps to relax the body and reduces stress, thus improving blood pressure. It increases serotonin output, lifting a client's mood. It is known to provide relief from headaches and twisted or injured muscles and to release rigid shoulders and necks.

## How it Works

The first recorded mention of massage in general, comes from ancient Greece and Egypt. It was used to heal the body. Deep tissue massage was frequently used for individual who were not helped by regular massage, but no guidelines were developed until the mid 1900s. Canadian doctor, Therese Phimmer, wrote a book on the subject in 1949 entitled "Muscles – Your Invisible Bonds." It served as the manual for deep tissue massage. She was able to cure the paralysis in her own legs using the method and opened a clinic in 1949.

Recipients might feel a bit stiff and have some minor pain issues up to two days after the massage. The only problem with the suction cups is that clients can get something that looks like a "hickey" from them.

As with any massage, avoid a heavy meal beforehand and drink water and other hydrating fluids both before and after the massage. Toxins are released by this treatment and water will help to flush them from the body. If you don't hydrate adequately, you may suffer greater soreness and stiffness than usual for a few days. Avoid strenuous activity after a deep tissue massage, but light stretching techniques can facilitate your body's recovery.

In a deep tissue massage, oil is used to allow the therapist's hands to move freely over the body. The hands, fingertips, knuckles, forearms and sometimes the elbows are used to accomplish treatment.

You will experience greater pressure on your body than in Swedish massage. The therapist utilizes body weight to lean into your muscles  The thumbs and fingertips of the therapist inspect and probe muscles and the areas in between them. If a knot is discovered, great pressure is applied and the fingers actually sink into the skin.

A knot consists of an adhesion made up of bands of rigid tissue. It forms as your body heals from an injury or as the result of sustained or increasing tension in your muscles, ligaments or tendons. These adhesions inhibit circulation and generate pain, which can reduce your range of motion.

In deep tissue massage, a knot is not smoothed away, but is pressed until it releases. This therapy may feel uncomfortable, but it should not cause terrible pain.

The natural reflex of a muscle is to resist pressure. If too much pressure is applied, the muscle will only tighten further. A skilled professional will know when to apply the correct amount of pressure to cause the muscle to relax instead of tensing further.

## Techniques

**Active Motion** includes the recipient in flexing and stretching muscles on which the therapist is applying pressure. When flexing, the fibers of the muscle spread, allowing the therapist to dig in deeply between them. The flexing motion also helps to minimize any pain you experience. This often takes 5 to 10 minutes to achieve, for a single muscle group.

**Passive Motion** – The therapist does all the work in passive motion, manipulating the muscle with one hand while moving the body part with the other. This is relaxing for the recipient but much more difficult for the therapist. An example would be moving the arm up and down from the shoulder while massaging the shoulder area.

**Static Pressure** – The therapist employs fingertips, thumbs, or elbows to administer pressure to points on the body. Static pressure, applied to a single muscle group, might take up to 20 minutes, because the pressure is applied very gradually and is released slowly as well.

**Muscle Stripping** – This is a rapid and aggressive movement on the muscle that can cause some pain. The therapist uses knuckles or an elbow to apply pressure and then strip or glide along the muscle while the recipient breathes deeply. This usually occurs in a single rapid motion although slow motion muscle stripping can be completed as well.

**Negative Pressure** involves the use of special suction cups. The suction cups are applied to the body, causing the muscle fibers to separate and expand as they are sucked into the cup. This creates some space between the muscle fibers and allows the toxins to flow out freely.

## Equipment

A massage table and heated oils are the essentials for this type of massage. The only additional equipment is a set of suction cups used for negative pressure techniques.

## Contraindications

Avoid deep tissue massage if you have an active infection, especially a skin infection, an open wound, or a rash. Do not participate in massage if you have recently undergone chemotherapy or radiation therapy. Check with a doctor first if you are prone to blood clots, have heart disease, or have osteoporosis.

Stay away from deep tissue massage if you are pregnant. A therapist will avoid the area of any hernias or tumors. Deep tissue massage therapists will not work on deep bruises and will avoid massaging in the vicinity of actively healing fractures.

# Chapter 4: Sports Massage

The origin of Sports Massage is Greece, the home of the Olympics, and Rome. Its evolution into a modern form of therapy included a runner from Finland, a doctor from Russia, and a German prisoner of war.

Although you would think that sports massage is only for athletes, it is actually for anyone; athlete or non-athlete. This therapy is especially useful for treating soft tissue injuries, but is also helpful for anyone who has issues with muscles, tendons or joints.

Sports massage can be employed to treat a specific injury. It is used mainly for athletes with sports-related injuries, but is also used as a preventative measure for individuals who practice highly repetitive movements. For example, baseball pitchers can wear down the rotator cuff due to overuse while pitching. Treating the shoulder via sports massage can keep a pitcher going for years without severe injury. At the same time, following rotator cuff surgery, an individual will benefit greatly from sports massage because it can speed the healing process.

Factory workers often use the same muscles to perform repeated motions, day in and day out. If, for example, assembly line workers screw mirrors on car doors all day long, the muscles in their wrists may be come fatigued. Sports massage can prevent fatigue-related injuries. It can also help workers recover from repetitive-motion injuries. Sports massage can also increase workers' range of motion, flexibility, and strength.

## Benefits

Anyone who overuses specific muscles will benefit greatly from sports massage. This therapy can condition muscles, tendons and connective tissues to tolerate increased use without injury. It can also help an individual recover from repetitive motion injuries.

Sports massage can reduce tension in muscles, arrest and reduce swelling, stop pain, and increase flexibility. It can improve the heart rate, lower blood pressure, increase circulation, and helps lymph fluids flow throughout the body.

The types of injuries sports medicine benefits are many. The list includes the dreaded tennis elbow, painful shin splints, corked thighs, hamstring injuries, sprains, strains, and contusions.

Sports massage is usually avoided until 48 hours have elapsed following an injury. Sometimes a bad sprain can take a week before the massage can take place. If there is bleeding at the site of the injury, massage must be avoided until any chance of bleeding has subsided.

## How it Works

The Romans and Greeks both improved the performance of their Olympic champions with massage, but the protocols in use today weren't employed until the 1924 Olympics. Paavo Nurmi was a successful Finnish runner who won five gold medals at the Olympic games that year. He attributed his success to a type of massage therapy he received in preparation for the Olympics.

Around the same time, a Russian doctor, I.M. Sarkoisof-Sirasin, began teaching methods of massage specially tailored to the needs of athletes. In 1945, Jack Meagher received a massage by a German prisoner of war that used a friction method. Jack believed his success in sports was in large part due to these massage techniques.

In 1970 James Cyriax, given the name of the father of orthopedic medicine, developed a similar technique and called it the deep friction method. He used it specifically to treat sports injuries. In 1985 the AMTA (The American Massage Therapy Association) began promoting a sports massage program, moving it to the forefront of massage protocols.

## Description

Many people who receive sports massage therapy attend a session every week or two. The techniques employed are similar to Swedish massage, along with the use of methods specific to the treatment of sports injuries.

Overuse of muscles can sometimes result in knots, which need to be relaxed in order for lactic acid to be released and for lymph liquids to flow properly through the body. Muscles are stretched, rubbed, and kneaded in order to promote this release, as well as to strengthen them, to increase their flexibility, and to reduce the chances of future injury. Following an injury, these same methods are employed to facilitate healing.

## Techniques

**Pumping** – The therapist stokes the damaged or tight muscle using more pressure at the beginning of the stroke. This creates a vacuum that propels fluid through the blood and the lymph vessels in the body.

**Deep Massage** – Deep massage opens up the pores in the muscles and allows fluids to be released. It causes lactic acid to flow out and promotes the influx of oxygen and other nutrients into the muscle. Deep massage can be a little painful, but it effectively helps muscles and their connective tissues become more flexible.

**Stretches** – In sports massage, the muscle is stretched lengthwise, which releases tension. Any type of sports training can cause the muscles, tendons, and the fascia surrounding the muscles to become hard and inflexible. Stretching softens up muscles and fascia and allows for both better mobility and increased circulatory flow throughout.

**Friction Massage** – Friction Massage is unique to sports massage. This technique helps tendons that might be slightly injured or stiff. It is also very useful to treat sprains. In this technique, the affected area is rubbed back and forth quickly to create friction. The friction stimulates the fibers of the tendon or muscles to unclump. Pressure is also applied, using the fingers and thumb to generate a pain that burns but should be bearable. If you feel no pain, the therapist is not working the right location.

Friction massage lasts for one to two minutes, until the sensitivity stops. The process is repeated until it stops hurting, followed by a third friction massage. At the end of this treatment, ice is applied for about two minutes, until the area becomes numb.

Many sports figures swear by this technique, saying it helps to heal injuries and enables them to finish out a game, in spite of injury.

**Equipment**

Oil is utilized to help fingers glide over muscles and tendons. A flat surface where the client can lie down is also a requirement. Many sports therapists employ the use of a variety of machines to help with the massage, as the situation warrants.

# Chapter 5: Trigger Point Massage

Trigger Point therapy has been employed in no less an auspicious venue than the American White House. At least two American presidents have benefitted from this form of therapy.

Fibers in the muscles, when used beyond the fatigue point, can pass beyond tension to stop functioning altogether, resulting in constant, debilitating pain. This pain can be alleviated by trigger point massage.

The purpose behind this type of massage is to reduce pain and "unknot" trigger points through cycles of targeted pressure and release. Deep breathing exercises are employed during treatment, primarily to manage the considerable pain inflicted in the process. However, any pain is worth it when the treatment deactivates trigger points and allows the muscles to function normally once more.

Trigger points are little knots of contracted muscle fibers that cause stiffness and soreness. Pain from these knots can radiate to other areas of the body. For example, when a knot is pressed in the forearm, your fingers may ache.

It takes a trained therapist to locate a trigger point and treat it. However, you can perform trigger point massage on your own body. This can actually be to your advantage, because you can inflict much more pain on yourself than you can bear receiving at the hands of another person.

It is not uncommon to require a few hours following treatment before a knot finally dissolves. Trigger points can cause pain, tingling and a numb feeling.

## Benefits

Trigger point massage is a non-invasive way to rid yourself of muscular pain. It is highly effective. People with pain in the back, legs, gluts, and feet often benefit the most from treatment. Trigger point therapy helps with shin splints, shoulder pain and rotator cuff injuries. It works wonders on migraines, sciatica, and low back pain and can bring some flexibility back to frozen shoulders. People with carpal tunnel, arthritis, muscle spasms, TMJ, and whiplash can also benefit from trigger point therapy, as can individuals suffering from menstrual cramps and muscle spasms.

## How it Works

The person most known for developing Trigger Point Massage is Dr. Janet Travell who served as personal physician for Presidents Kennedy and Johnson. She treated John F. Kennedy for pain that could have ended his political career.

At one point, Kennedy's lower back pain was radiating down his left leg, making it almost impossible for him to walk. Thanks to Dr. Travell's groundbreaking research into myofascial disorders, she was able to successfully treat Kennedy's condition and address its source. Credit for the "trigger point" moniker goes to Dr. Travell.

This method of massage actually dates back a little further, to the 1840s, but was not developed extensively until Dr. Travell popularized it, co-authoring several books about the methodology.

Trigger point massage consists primarily of applying heavy, pointed pressure directly atop a trigger point. Therapists explore the body with their fingers in order to locate activated trigger points. Then they apply pressure to cause it to dissolve. Therapists work on an area for anywhere from a few seconds to five minutes.

During treatment, the client lies in a comfortable position, but may not stay comfortable for long. Trigger point massage can be very painful, but the pain should never be unbearable. It may cause you to flinch or squirm. In some cases, you will feel radiating pain or pain referred to an entirely different part of the body, when the trigger is pressed.

The therapist begins with a moderate amount of pressure for a few seconds and only applies stronger pressure if the knot doesn't give way to lesser persuasion. Pressure is applied via the fingers, elbows or knuckles

Some therapists will inject an area with lidocaine to minimize the pain prior to performing the therapy. They may also probe knots with a dry needle, but the recipient always has the option of refusing this procedure. The good thing about trigger point massage is that the recipient usually realizes instant pain relief.

## Techniques

**Self-Massage** – Use your own fingertips and thumbs to find trigger points. The most effective tool you can have to perform this type of massage on yourself is a plain old tennis ball. Lie on a ball. Move back and forth over the ball, pausing at spots that are painful. You can work most of your body this way, using body weight to provide pressure to areas that are painful. This works really well with back, shoulder, and glut problems and will often help a stiff neck. For upper body areas, you can stand, placing the tennis ball between yourself and a wall, and lean into any sore spots.

**Compression** – Digital compression is the term used for compression of knots during trigger point massage. Therapists compress the trigger point until they feel a change in the knot. It may release completely and go away or it may feel mushier. They never sustain compression longer than 90 seconds at a time, but may return to a trigger point several times during a session.

**Kneading** – Therapists make small circular kneading strokes on the area, traveling in the direction of the muscle fibers. This can give clients a rest from the application of pressure and grant the therapist a breather, but it also helps break down knots.

## Equipment

You will need a place to lie down. A therapist will often provide a treatment bed. No oil is used and clients can be fully clothed. A plain old tennis ball is often all that is needed for self treatment.

The <u>Back Pain Power Bar</u> by ProMajestic and the <u>Backnobber II</u> by the Pressure Positive Company are simple tools that can facilitate self-treatment. They help you target and treat otherwise hard-to-reach trigger points.

## Contraindications

Avoid trigger point massage if you have any type of infectious illness. Do not participate in the massage if you have open sores, bruising or recent injuries. It is best to wait at least a few days to a week before treating a fresh injury using this modality. Avoid trigger point massage when you are taking blood thinners.

Most recipients come away with some bruising, so the trigger point area can be a little sensitive for a few days. To reduce the tenderness following treatment, take a long soak in an Epsom salts bath.

After you have received treatment, it is very important to stay hydrated in the days that follow. The breakdown of trigger points releases toxins into your bloodstream and water helps to flush them out.

# Chapter 6: Thai Massage

Thai massage originates, as one might assume, in Thailand, but its current form includes a mix of methods from India and South Asia.

Thai Massage is different from other massage methods; it is also called Thai Yoga because the therapist uses his own hands, legs, feet, and knees to move the client into a variety of yoga-like positions and stretches. Because the therapist does all the positioning work, it is also known as "the lazy man's yoga" or "yoga without any work."

There are two basic styles of Thai massage. One is a traditional and ancient form practiced around Nepal and the northern regions of India. It is called "Nuat Phan Boran." This form of Thai massage starts out with meditation involving both the therapist and the recipient. The second type is a more modern massage form that may forgo the meditation and start right in on the massage; it is called "Nuat Phan Thai".

The theory behind this methodology is that all forms of life are driven by a vital force called lom. Lom is carried through the body along pathways called sen. It is believed that disease and illness are caused when the sen becomes blocked or injured. Massage frees the trapped lom and stimulates its flow so that the body returns to balance.

Thai Massage only recently grew beyond the country's borders. It has only been widely practiced in the West for the past 15 years or so. Sessions are usually individualized for the client and the specific treatment depends on the blockages that are encountered.

## Benefits

Thai massage accomplishes much of what other massage modalities pursue. It relaxes the body, reduces stress, increases circulation, activates more energy, and increases both range of motion and flexibility. It also centers an individual's body, mind, and soul. It helps to detoxify the body and boost the immune system. Thai massage promotes breathing and works to realign the body. It calms arthritis and helps athletes perform better. The massage benefits muscles by strengthening them.

Thai massage has been found to improve creativity and help with concentration, thanks to meditation and breathing exercises performed both prior to and during the massage. Through Thai Massage, recipients often develop a sense of discipline and increased self-control.

## How it Works

Thai massage was developed by Buddha's physician, Jivaka Kumar, about 2,500 years ago. It incorporates a bit of Chinese medicine and is similar to working with meridians. The massage techniques are based on a mixture of theologies from India and other Southeast Asian cultures. The Indian Ayurvedic principals weigh heavily and sometimes acupressure is used in addition to energy balancing techniques.

## Description

Thai massage is usually performed on a padded mat placed on the floor. No oil is used on the body and the recipient and therapist are fully clothed. There is consistent body contact between therapist and recipient most of the time. While other forms of massage employ rubbing or kneading of the muscles, Thai massage compresses, stretches, pulls and rocks the muscles via the motions of the therapist. The only pressure applied to muscles is deep static or rhythmic pressure.

During a massage session – which may last for two hours – you can expect the therapist to pull and crack fingers, toes and knuckles. The idea is that, while there are 10 basic sen lines, there are 72,000 sen lines running throughout your body. The therapist's work removes any blockages that prevent the life force, or lom, from flowing freely and being evenly distributed throughout the body.

Deep rhythmical beating is performed by both therapist and recipient, as is mindfulness or the awareness of the breath. The therapist may give the recipient a mantra to concentrate on before beginning and may focus on loving kindness and compassion. While this is going on, each sen is pressed in every direction by adjusting the client's positioning. The client's part throughout the massage is to concentrate on breathing and sustaining any mantra or visualization requested by the therapist.

## Techniques

Two main techniques are employed during Thai massage. **Compressions** involve pressing on parts of the body. The therapist exerts pressure as needed on soft tissues and applies pressure in every direction.

**Stretches** start out small, but may be extended very far. Each muscle is stretched as well as the related joints. The therapist will stretch further than the recipient would ever be able to accomplish by themselves.

In our daily life, our muscles tend to shorten, thanks to our activities and the various stresses we face. Thai massage stretches the muscles to where they should be, restoring their normal, healthy state upon awakening. Shortened muscles tend to block the lom from moving through the body.

The therapist also places the recipient in several yoga poses and asks them to continue meditating and breathing. It is surprising how everything relaxes and mobility returns.

## Contraindications

You should avoid Thai massage if you have any skin irritations or open wounds. Wait until they heal before participating in massage. Individuals who are prone to blood clots should participate with care, as should anyone with heart problems, bruises, tumors, hernias, and those who are pregnant.

## Equipment

The only equipment that is necessary for Thai massage is a low padded mat. The therapist will clean the pad with antibacterial wipes prior to the session.

# Chapter 7: Neuromuscular Massage

Neuromuscular massage developed in two places simultaneously, without one knowing about the other. The two origins are the United States and Europe.

Neuromuscular massage is more of a therapeutic treatment than traditional massage. It is similar to Deep Tissue and Trigger Point massage, but includes more emphasis on knowledge of the body's central nervous system. Therapists are trained in the effects of the nervous system on the muscles, tendons and connective tissues, along with a basic understanding of the skeletal system. They use pressure on specific points and deeply manipulate soft tissue with the goal of balancing out the nervous system to alleviate pain.

## Benefits

Neuromuscular massage helps to balance the nervous system, which includes the spinal column, the brain, and all the nerves running through the body. The treatment is specialized for the control of pain. Those who benefit from treatment include individuals with sciatica, rotator cuff problems, TMJ, carpal tunnel and migraines. The massage techniques help victims of trauma or individuals suffering from soft tissue injuries and treats muscle spasms.

This treatment has been known to improve chronic neck and back pain, strains, stiffness of joints, whiplash, and hip, knee, or ankle pain. It restores flexibility and releases endorphins into the body. Endorphins are the body's natural painkillers, so this treatment offers a holistic approach to pain management that can minimize the need for prescription medication.

## How it Works

Neuromuscular massage is about 60 years old and goes back to the mid 1930s. Stanley Lief, from Latvia, was a student of Ayurvedic medicine in India but was also skilled in chiropractic and osteopathic techniques. In 1925, he moved from Latvia to Europe and began to perform neuromuscular therapy with his cousin, Boris Chaitow. Stanley's son, Peter, developed many of the therapies that are in use today.

Raymond Nimmo was a 1931 graduate of the Palmer School in the United States. He developed some of the same ideas as Lief, taking Trigger Point therapy a little further, pairing it with the study of the nervous system, and developing additional procedures that are in use today.

## Description

Neuromuscular massage has several objectives. One is to improve the blood flow to muscles, tendons and connective tissues. When the blood is not flowing freely, oxygen levels are low in the soft tissues. This causes lactic acid to build up, creating muscle soreness. Often muscles tie up in knots that inhibit blood flow

Another objective of neuromuscular massage is to remove knots from the muscles. Nerves tend to become trapped by bone, cartilage or soft tissue. A common example is when the sciatic nerve is out of place. Neuromuscular massage helps to untrap those nerves.

A secondary goal is to balance the skeletal system so that nerves are less likely to be impinged and muscles remain knot-free. Bad posture is often addressed as well as proper lifting technique. The primary difference between deep tissue and trigger point massage is that both the nervous and skeletal systems are involved in the massage as well as in preventative techniques. The client is instructed in ways to prevent future pain by changing posture and movements.

## Techniques

**Pressure** is applied to the muscles with fingers, knuckles and elbows. The amount of pressure used depends on the need, but it may be uncomfortably painful. Pressure is applied for 10 to 30 seconds, until the muscle starts to relax. The therapist moves the skin toward the painful area while applying pressure.

**Stroking** movements are also used. These movements relax the muscles further and promote blood circulation.

**Stretching** – Often, when a nerve is compressed, stretching can help to work it free. Therapists will locate the pinched nerve by examining a client's range of motion and strength levels. They then use resisted stretch techniques to accomplish relief. Resisted stretching carries the muscles far beyond what is normal, but remains within safe boundaries.

**Other Issues** – The therapist is not necessarily limited to massage techniques. Other issues are also considered with pain resolution as the goal. A therapist may look at your posture and give you exercises and tips to resolve your problem by realigning your skeletal system.

A therapist may pay attention to life activities that impact your skeletal alignment. Nutrition may also be addressed. Our cells are weakened by not getting the nutrients they need, potentially causing pain. Good nutrition is one of the keys to making your body pain-free.

## Contraindications

People with congestive heart failure or kidney failure should avoid neuromuscular massage, as should individuals with phlebitis, blood clot issues, bleeding disorders, or cellulitis. If you have a skin condition or are fighting cancer, you should check with your doctor before proceeding with this type of therapy.

**Equipment**

Neuromuscular massage takes place on a flat surface. Oils and lotions are sometimes used but are not always required.

# Chapter 8: Chair Massage

Chair massage is a popular trend that began in San Francisco. David Palmer, head of TouchPro Institute in San Francisco in the 1980s, is often referred to as "The Father of Chair Massage."

Palmer invented the portable chair after coming across some ancient Japanese block prints of people sitting on stools while being massaged. This gave him the idea for a more comfortable massage venue that allowed the client to be treated in a relaxed, informal setting.

Palmer's chair causes the recipient to lean forward and cradles the face in an open cushioned face rest. The treatment employed during chair massage is a Japanese form called Amma. Amma is a deep tissue massage that uses acupressure, stroking, and percussion methods.

Starting from this point, David Palmer developed a light massage method performed in a chair that could be easily embraced by the masses. Among early clients, he was commissioned by Apple Computers to visit their workplace periodically to offer chair massages to employees. The purpose was to relieve job-related stress so that individuals would feel happier and be more productive on the job.

This is probably one of the most accessible and affordable types of massage. If you are new to massage, this is an ideal place to start.

You can find opportunities for a chair massage at malls, airports, and fairs. Some companies bring in chair massage therapists on a regular basis to increase the productivity of their employees.

Chair massage is designed to relax muscles and improve circulation in the body. That is all. It is *not* designed to relieve pain or treat injuries, although these may be helped in the process.

The practitioner provides a portable chair that seats the client leaning forward with support for the head. Sessions run from 15 to 30 minutes. This makes it possible for busy workers to enjoy a quick massage during a coffee break or over the lunch break. The client is fully clothed and the massage is accomplished without the use of oils, which would only mess up the clothing.

Chair massage is not considered therapeutic per se. While individuals who perform the massage may hold certification in one or more forms of massage therapy, certification is not required in this case, so sometimes you will hear massage providers referred to as practitioners, instead of therapists.

The recipient indicates what parts of the body need a massage. The massage may be addressed to the head and face, legs, feet, arms, hands, shoulders, and the spine. The purpose of this massage is to relax and reinvigorate the client.

## Benefits

Some organizations that provide chair massages for their employees cite multiple benefits. They report reduced stress, improved circulation, and more relaxed workers. Chair massage can also decrease blood pressure and heart rate, a boon for high-stress jobs. Workers are also reported to be more productive and happier following a massage.

## How it Works

The client sits or kneels comfortably on the special chair, leaning forward. The face is cradled in a cushioned headrest that allows one to breathe freely while appropriately supporting the neck. The therapist massages the head and neck, working down into the shoulders, arms, and hands. A massage may include the upper and lower back. No oil is used and clients are fully clothed throughout.

## Techniques

The techniques for chair massage are the same as for many other types of massage including petrissage, kneading and percussion as in Swedish massage.

**Shoulder Techniques** – Kneading is the method used to relax shoulders, arms and hands. Tension seems to settle there because of sitting at a computer for hours at a time. Practitioners start at the base of the neck and gently squeeze and knead the shoulder muscles, working toward the shoulder and the arms. They may move back and forth three or four times. The hands can also be kneaded gently, which reduces fatigue caused by sustained bouts of typing.

**Neck Techniques** – Stroking is the method best used on the neck area. Beginning at the base of the neck, the practitioner traces circular strokes going up the neck back on both sides using thumbs or fingers.

**Upper Back Techniques**- Percussion works best on larger areas, like the back. The practitioner may use either the sides or the heels of the hands, tapping rhythmically up and down. The tapping will begin lightly and grow stronger. Percussion is never applied directly onto the spine or near the kidneys, but is great for the upper back.

**Lower Back Techniques** – Pressure works well on the lower back and sometimes on the shoulders. The practitioner applies hands and leans body weight into the muscle. Pressure increases slowly and is released gradually. Therapists use their own body weight to apply pressure.

## Equipment

Chair massage requires the use of a portable chair. These are usually collapsible and lightweight, making them easily transported to various sites. The chair is adjustable to fit the size of any client. Some therapists also incorporate the use of relaxing sounds and scents, but these are not required.

The therapist will bring sanitizer to cleanse the chair following each massage and disposable coverings for the face rest, to prevent clients from transferring bacteria.

## Contraindications

Individuals with hypertension, diabetes, cancer, recent fractures or herniated discs should avoid chair massage. If you experience numbness or a tingling sensation in your hands and feet on a regular basis, you also avoid this therapy. Remember that not all practitioners will have the medical background required by other massage modalities; they may not be equipped to identify and treat specific ailments

There should be no negative side effects to chair massage because it is a light touch therapy. The only danger is slight bruising or soreness for those who are not at all accustomed to receiving massage therapy. Sanitary measures are commonly practiced to prevent the transmission of germs. However, if you have not seen the chair wiped down before you approach, feel free to ask the practitioner to clean the chair.

Diabetics may experience low sugar levels following any massage. Anyone allergic to vinyl or leather should avoid direct contact with the chair and the face rest.

Chair massage is a great way to help staff reduce stress and increase productivity on the job. Research shows that employees focus much better if they are treated to a chair massage; it also makes them feel like their company really cares. This is a luxury offered in the workplace, to shoppers in a mall, or to an individual who has been stuffed into the small passenger seat of an airplane for hours. Chair massage is much more affordable and much less intimidating than other types of massage.

# Chapter 9: Hot Stone Massage

Hot Stone massage was first reported in China, but was not limited to that country. The Native Americans and Polynesians have also used hot stone treatment.

Hot Stone Massage incorporates some of the elements of both Swedish massage and deep tissue massage. The stones used in this form of therapy are smooth river rocks that are heated and held in the therapist's hands or placed on targeted areas of the body to release their heat deep into tight muscles. Recipients have remarked on the comforting feeling of the heat that helps them relax.

This form of massage is well suited for people with serious muscle tension who do not respond well to deep tissue massage. The heat penetrates deeply into muscles, encouraging them to relax. The heat also increases circulation by expanding the blood vessels. The result is a slightly sedative effect.

A hot stone massage can take anywhere from one hour to 90 minutes, but its benefits are long-lasting

## Benefits

Arthritis and osteoarthritis sufferers find that hot stone massage helps them greatly. It also helps individuals with chronic back or shoulder pain. Fibromyalgia sufferers may experience pain relief and the heat from the stones can calm muscle spasms.

If you have reduced circulation, this treatment will expand your arteries and veins to increase blood flow. Insomniacs may find they sleep better after a session and hot stone massage can even improve symptoms of depression and anxiety.

## The Origin of Hot Stone Massage

Over 2000 years ago, the Chinese used hot stones to help organs in the body function more effectively. Native Americans used hot stones to treat sore muscles and stones have long been used to heat the sweat lodge, a place for physical purification and spiritual enlightenment. Many years ago in Hawaii, healers wrapped smooth hot stones in large leaves and placed them on areas of the body that were unusually sore. In this case, the stones they employed were volcanic and were also rubbed all over the body.

In the early 1990s, Mary Nelson, a resident of Tucson Arizona, developed what she called LaStone Therapy, after visiting a sauna and noticing that they used stones to heat the room. Following a vision from her Native American spirit guide who explained their use, she began to incorporate hot stones into her therapeutic practice.

## The Stones

Stones of varying sizes are employed in hot stone massage. Larger stones are used on larger muscles, while smaller stones are used to treat hands, feet, arms, and lower legs. The preferred composition is basalt, which consists of black volcanic rock. These stones absorb heat well and radiate it much longer than other types of stone. They are somewhat flat and very smooth.

In most cases, an electric warmer filled with water is used to heat the stones to between 120 and 150 degrees F.

## The Treatment

The person being massaged lies face down on a therapy table. The therapist may begin to warm up the client's body with a little Swedish massage, oiling the body to facilitate the movement of both hands and stones. Following the warm-up, stones are placed along the spine, in the client's hands and between the toes in order to enhance the flow of circulation. After these stones have done their duty, they are removed and the therapist grasps freshly heated stones, using them to massage the client's body.

Cold marble stones may also be applied strategically to strengthen cellular structure and draw inflammation out of muscles. Cool marine stones are used to infuse a variety of minerals into the body and can be used to help the body repair damaged capillaries while promoting relaxation.

## Techniques

There are no set techniques of hot stone massage, although stone placement is informed by the location of various chakras. Therapists learn by experience which stones are most effective to treat specific needs. Most individuals will use a circular motion or an up and down sliding motion when massaging with stone in hand.

Sometimes stones used to massage the body are colored to match the different chakras:

- The chakra associated with red is at the base of the spine and is associated with energy in the body. A garnet might be used to massage the bottom of the back to the buttocks. This is the base chakra.

- The chakra at the naval is associated with the color orange and is considered the seat of sexuality and creativity. Carnelian is often used to massage the belly and the hip area.

- Yellow is the color of the chakra at the solar plexus. Citrine or topaz is used to improve energy to the nervous system. The mid back, the stomach near the diaphragm, and the lungs are massaged with this stone.

- It is no surprise that the love chakra is found at the center of the chest where your heart is located. Stones employed here are pink or green and are used on the chest and the back in the chest. Rose quartz and jade are the stones of choice for this chakra.

- Communication is the main goal of the throat chakra. The corresponding color is blue and its stone is aquamarine.

- The third eye, situated in the forehead between the two physical eyes, represents the next chakra. It rules the intuition and its associated color is dark blue. Lapis is the stone used to stimulate this chakra.

- The top of the head, or the crown, is the final chakra. It is associated with spirituality and its color is violet. Amethyst is the stone of choice here.

It is interesting that gemstones are usually angular, not smooth. Although some therapists use tumbled stones in massage modalities, others prefer to use the stones in their natural state. In this case, treatment consists of laying them on the spine near the focus of the chakra while performing massage with other, smoother stones.

## Equipment

Therapy is performed on a table or other flat surface that has a horseshoe headrest for prone treatment. Oils are used to allow the stones to move seamlessly across the skin. Sheets and other linens are used to cover the parts of the body not undergoing treatment. Sanitizing solutions are used to disinfect the rocks every time they are used.

## Contraindications

Some people have skin that does not tolerate direct heat well, so they should avoid hot stone massage.

In treatment, usually some sort of barrier is placed between the skin and the stones. While stones are never subjected to extreme heat, there is always the chance of being burned when the stones are placed directly on the skin and allowed to set there for a while. A thin towel can ensure that your skin is safe from too much heat. When a therapist is manipulating the stones over your body, there is less opportunity for excessive heat exposure; nevertheless, speak up if at any time the stones feel too hot.

Avoid treatment if you have a contagious disease or skin lesions. The stones are always sanitized, but for your own health it is best to forego treatment until your condition improves.

Individuals with varicose veins, edema, or high blood pressure should avoid hot stone treatment. The heat causes your blood vessels to expand and this can cause harm if you have any of these conditions.

Your therapist will avoid areas of bruising or open wounds, but it is wise to point out these areas at the start of a session.

If you are pregnant, only subject yourself to hot stone massage at the hand of a therapist trained in treating women during pregnancy. Children under the age of 18 should never be treated with this modality, because of their greater skin sensitivity. Individuals beyond the age of 60 often have thinner skin that would be easily injured by the application of hot stones, so they are wise to avoid this treatment as well.

If you have circulatory problems or a heart condition and still want to try hot stone massage, first discuss this treatment with your physician. A professional massage therapist is able to take precautions that can prevent you from being in danger while ensuring you receive the benefits of hot stone treatment.

If your immune system is in any way compromised, you must insist on knowing both how the stones are heated and what measures are taken to prevent infection. For all people, appropriate heat levels and the minimization of bacterial transmission are important. Any therapist should have a clear protocol in place for sanitizing the stones between clients. Bacteria can be easily passed from the stones to your body and the chance of infection is only amplified by the presence of heat, so appropriate precautions are a must.

# Chapter 10: Erotic Massage

It is hard to pin down the origin of Erotic massage, as the subject has been shrouded in the mists of taboo for many years. However, the practice of treating women for issues of "hysteria" and "womb disease" by incorporating aspects of erotic massage has been in use since before the 1650s, when Pieter van Foreest, a Dutchman, began to write about it. Nonetheless, erotic massage didn't just start in the 17th century. A cursory glance at the Kama Sutra, which emerged in India during the 10th century, will confirm its earlier presence.

You may think erotic massage is a forbidden practice – and it is illegal in some states, provinces and countries – but the practice is a viable treatment for certain dysfunctions. Erotic massage is defined as a technique applied to another person's erogenous zones in order to create sexual excitement and arousal. It doesn't necessarily end in orgasm. This type of massage contains some health and emotional benefits, yet because of its connection to sexuality, the treatment has garnered a negative reputation.

While other forms of massage may elicit sexual pleasure, that is not their focus; this result, however, is the primary purpose of erotic massage. Many sex therapists apply erotic massage as a treatment modality to help recipients release stress and relax, while fostering increased body awareness. Therapists do not usually participate in the therapy itself, but instead instruct bonded couples in the practice.

There is a fine line between massage and prostitution, so fine in fact that many American states consider it illegal to engage in sexual touch. It is permissible in Holland, Australia, Canada, New Zealand, Romania, Thailand, Japan, and in some areas of the United Kingdom. In most countries, however, erotic massage is considered legal between consenting adults, when practiced within their own home.

## Benefits

There are several benefits to erotic massage. Men who experience consistent premature ejaculation can be helped by using the techniques of erotic massage to release stress and reduce anxiety. Erotic massage regulates the blood flow, relaxes muscles and generally awakens the senses of both male and female. Emotionally, it can bring couples closer together, improving their relational connection while enhancing the physical and sexual relationship. It can also result in improved confidence in social interactions.

## How it Works

The history of erotic massage is interesting, to say the least. During the 17th century, women were often afflicted with something called hysteria. Once a prescription for genital massage was given them, their temperament improved markedly. This massage was performed by either a midwife or a physician. There was absolutely no risk involved in the treatment. Anyone who performed the service became quite popular; women would frequently request treatment. It made the clients happy and the midwife or doctor wealthy.

Manipulation often took some time to accomplish the desired result, so the husbands would sometimes be employed to assist. When vibrators came into existence, treatment became much easier and faster.

Vibrator-assisted treatment was first used in doctors' offices and in asylums, especially in France. The advent of electricity in the home made vibrators increasingly accessible. Popular use grew and the modality was considered quite acceptable at the time, because it was viewed as a form of medical treatment.

Hydro-treatment, the use of water to achieve orgasm, came into play during the 1870s. Men were out of luck though, because this treatment only applied to women.

## Description

Erotic Massage consists of physical touch around the erogenous zones with the primary aim of arousal. In other types of massage, the aim is to treat health issues or to alleviate pain. With erotic massage however, the purpose is to help the body relax through pleasure; and any other health benefits are secondary in nature.

This therapy is designed primarily for couples and doesn't always end in intercourse, but this is a frequent "byproduct." Regular sessions of sexual massage tend to relax the pelvic region and help participants work together to prolong their arousal. Partners take turns receiving and then giving erotic massage. Both partners are naked throughout the session and oils are used as a sensual aid. Oils help fingers slide on the skin and enhance an individual's sensitivity to touch. Some oils are specifically formulated for erotic massage; other oils may compromise condoms and may limit the effectiveness of other birth control methods as well.

## Techniques

Many of the techniques employed during erotic massage are similar to those of other massage techniques. They are described below:

**Kneading** can be relaxing, but it can also stimulate. It consists of grabbing a handful of flesh and gently squeezing it with the fingers and hands while pushing rapidly into the body. Kneading is most useful on the back, shoulders, belly, buttocks, thighs, calf muscles and upper arms.

**Hacking** employs the outside edges of the hands and the action looks like performing light karate chops to the body. It pulls blood toward the surface of the skin. This technique works well on the shoulders, back, buttocks and the back of the thighs.

**Friction** consists of rubbing the hands rapidly against the skin's surface. This creates heat that helps to permeate muscles. Friction should only be applied to less sensitive areas of the body. These include the back, buttocks and shoulders.

**Knuckling** consists of using the knuckles to grind into tight muscles, twisting to loosen them. It is most effective when applied to the spine, buttocks, the back of legs, the thighs, the base of the neck, and the arches of the feet.

**Draining** is a deep pressure technique applied to muscles. It consists of holding a partner's arm at the wrist and then, with the other thumb on the inside of the arm, sliding the thumb from shoulder to elbow. You then use the flat of your hand, sliding it down the inside of the arm. The same motion can be performed along the back of the calf, while holding the ankle.

**Cupping** is accomplished by rounding – or cupping – the hands over the skin and pounding as if drumming with alternating hands. It is applied to fleshy areas on the calves, thighs, back and buttocks.

Erotic massage is most effective when you alternate between the more strenuous techniques described above and the lighter touches described here. These gentler techniques also lend themselves to promoting arousal.

**Stroking** uses the tips of the fingers to lightly touch the skin in long strokes. Use this technique on the back, sides, shoulders, arms, buttocks, legs, chest, breasts or stomach.

**Feathering** is similar to stroking except you use one hand after the other in a rapid succession of stroking motions. This can be used anywhere on the body from the top of the head to the feet, including the erogenous zones

**Flowing** – Your hands lie flat and sweep in long, smooth movements along the curves of the body. It is important to keep the hands well-oiled so they will slide easily, without any distracting stuttering.

**Circling** – consists of making little circles on your partner's skin, moving your hands apart back together again. The touch is light, yet enough pressure should be exerted to allow the circles to be felt. Perform circling on the belly, chest, breasts, thighs, or buttocks. The breasts, along with the front and sides of the neck respond well to very tiny circles while the back, shoulders, belly and thighs lend themselves well to larger circles.

The following are more sensual techniques applied to or affecting the breasts, vagina or penis.

**Rocking** – Rocking stimulates the genital area as the whole body moves along the bed. With your partner lying face down, begin by rocking the hips back and forth, then up and down, applying pressure lightly to the pelvis.

**Licking and Biting** – You can use the tip of the tongue in some areas and keep it flat in others for variety. This works well on the neck, face, breasts or chest, as well as on the vaginal area and the penis. Nibble gently with your teeth, but avoid inflicting pain. Biting can cause great arousal almost anywhere on the body.

**Manual Stimulation** – Manual stimulation using the fingers or the whole hand is all part of erotic massage. There are many ways to achieve this using circling and stroking in the erogenous zones.

The idea is to keep your partner guessing as to what is next. You may start with some kneading on the back all the way down to the buttocks, then switch to feathering and ending with a little rocking or licking. Then try some other techniques ranging from greater pressure to light stroking to manual stimulation.

## Contraindications

You should only avoid erotic massage if you have any condition, determined by your physician, that renders you unsuitable for sex.

## Equipment

The obvious equipment is a bed, but fragrances to scent the room, and oils with pleasing aromas are also appropriate for erotic massage. You may also want to bring some sex toys to play with.

Take erotic massage slow and easy. Start gently and build with more pressure. Encourage breathing heavily and in unison. Attempt to keep the arousal going for a while before orgasm is achieved. Some couples even find it satisfying to enjoy multiple orgasms during the massage. The course of the massage and the depth of erotic pleasure experienced are only limited by what you and your partner prefer and by what you both want from the massage.

# Chapter 11: Tantric Massage

The tantric methods originate in ancient India, based on the deity named Shiva and his lover, Shakti. The technique of tantra has been in use for over 5,000 years and may be found in the ancient texts of the Kama Sutra. This practice is said to enhance health and well-being for those who participate in it.

Tantric massage uses sexual energy in order to heal and help participants bring themselves to a higher state of consciousness. It is designed to connect the body with the mind and soul of each person and then connect these to the other participant.

This is erotic massage, with a twist. All parts of the body are massaged so that energy flows throughout the individual's body as well as from one participant to the other. Orgasm is not a goal of tantric massage. In fact, many who perform tantric massage never experience orgasm, neither during nor following a therapy session. At the same time, some partners do engage in intercourse at the end of a session, but only after holding off a climax for an extended period of time.

Tantric massage is said to connect partners in ways that go beyond normal sex. Partners move together, breathe together, and some say their hearts beat in unison during a massage.

## Benefits

Tantric massage heightens awareness of one's body. Participants often eat better and are motivated to exercise to keep their bodies in shape as a result. They may sleep better, breathe deeper, relax more fully and find themselves more frequently at peace.

Tantric massage helps to invigorate a low libido and can relieve physical pain or emotional anxiety. It may also lessen the effects of stress. Men with premature ejaculation often receive help through tantric techniques, as do women who have a difficulty achieving orgasm.

## Origins

The word "Tantra" comes from a Sanskrit term meaning to manifest, expand or to put forth. The massage is said to expand awareness; you do expend great amounts of energy during the massage.

The seven chakras are integral to Tantric massage. Tantric massage involves "spinning" the chakras, a process which awakens the Kundalini, a mythical serpent that rises from the base of the spine to heal the body. The god Shiva and his lover Shakti are said to have developed this massage around 5,000 years ago.

## How It Works

In tantric massage, there are periods of activity and movement and periods of rest or peaceful silence. The stimulation produced by the massage encourages transcendence by the participants; it brings them to the point where nothing else matters but the strong erotic sensations they are experiencing.

Participants are naked throughout a session. The hands and fingers move all over the body in this form of massage. Touches start very light and become progressively stronger and faster.

Scented oils are frequently used to enhance the experience.

## Techniques

**Meditation** – It is a tradition to begin a tantric session with meditation. Namaste means, "I honor the Divine within you." Participants sit or kneel facing each other with hands pressed together before their chests and elbows bent. Each participant reflects on what the other person means to him or her, then waits for the partner to finish before closing eyes, bowing heads, and speaking "namaste" to each other.

**Unison Breathing** – During meditation, partners breathe in unison.

**Pranayama breathing** is a technique employed to cause the Kundalini to rise up the spine. It also prevents orgasm from occurring. Air is puffed through the mouth while pulling in the stomach muscles sharply. The stomach must relax before the next breath is taken. This changes the blood chemistry of the male; it stops blood from flowing to the penis and arrests orgasm.

This process can also serve the female partner. When sexually aroused, the breath naturally quickens and becomes irregular. Pranayama breathing is purposeful, slow, even, and balanced. Breaths are long. When one partner breathes in the other is breathing out, matching a visualization of ocean waves lapping the shore and then retreating.

**Hand Slide** – You use your hand to slide up and down the body. Slide up and down on either side of the spine, traveling from neck to buttocks, then up over the shoulders, and down again. In a second movement, you move up the neck, then over the shoulder and down the arms to the fingers. Oil is used to facilitate this technique.

**Pull Up Stroking** – Placing the hand over one hip, gently pull the flesh up toward the spine. Do the same with the other hip, then each side of the waist. Pull one side of the chest/breast toward the spine and then the other side. All movements are performed gently.

**Kneading** – Knead the shoulders, back, buttocks, arms and legs much as you would in Swedish massage.

**Feather Stroke** – Use the fingertips with very light fluttery motions anywhere on the body.

**Resting Positions** – All the activity in tantric massage periodically calls for a break  There are two resting positions used to keep in contact with your partner. The first is to lie on your back with your hands touching the feet of your partner in a star-like configuration.  This position will ground partners.

The other rest pose is called the Yab-yum position where the male sits cross-legged and the woman sits in his lap facing him with legs wrapped around his waist.  It is suggested that this position be used when you rest, unless both partners wish to engage in intercourse, which can also be performed in this position.

**Chakra Spinning** – There are seven chakras as follows:

1.  The base or root chakra influences sex and survival and is positioned at the base of the spine, at the tailbone.

2.  The sacral chakra influences emotions and sensuality and is found two inches below the navel.

3.  The Solar Plexus chakra guides truth and ego and is positioned near the stomach in the upper abdomen.

4.  The Heart chakra guides love and sacredness.  It is located in the center of the chest above the heart.

5.  The Throat chakra influences communication and creativity.  It is located in the throat area.

6.  The third eye chakra is the source of intuition and wisdom.  It is located between the eyes above the bridge of the nose.

7.  The Crown chakra is also known as the bliss chakra.  It is located on the top of the head

The following are techniques for stimulating these chakras to spin, which is one of the goals of tantric massage.

1.  Use two fingers in a circular motion near the pubic hairline.  When rest is needed, lay the hand flat on the area, and then begin again.

2. Use two fingers in a circular motion on the belly. Rest as needed in the same way as before.

3. Use two fingers in a circular motion at the top of the stomach below the ribs.

4. Use two fingers in circular motions between the breasts, then rest.

5. Use two fingers in light circular motions at the throat, avoiding the Adam's apple, then rest as needed.

6. Use two fingers in circular motion between the eyebrows, then rest. Do not use oil here.

7. To stimulate the crown chakra place one hand on the crown of the head and the other on the penis or vagina and do not move. Just apply gentle pressure to both. No oil is used here, either.

Move in clockwise circles to excite and spin the chakras. Perform some massage, some rest, and some chakra work, and then let your partner take a turn.

## Contraindications

Contagious skin conditions can be dangerous to the partner as can the flu or a cold. Be careful with inflammatory issues like arthritis. Blood clots may also be dislodged by tantric massage.

Avoid any type of oil in the genital area and use only lubricants that have been specially formulated for those areas.

## Equipment

The only things needed for tantric massage are oils and a bed.

In this form of massage, whatever works for you and your partner is fine. You may or may not want to have sex following a massage. Awakening the Kundalini can be extremely satisfying in itself and you may choose to withhold orgasm for hours or days following a massage.

# Chapter 12: Aromatherapy Massage

Essential oils have been extracted for therapeutic use since the Middle Ages, growing out of the practice, from antiquity, of using certain plants to heal illnesses. The term "aromatherapy" was coined by French chemist, René Gattefossé, in the early 1900s.

Modern usage in the West began when Gattefossé burned his arm in his laboratory and plunged it into the closest liquid available, a vat of lavender oil. When the burn healed quicker than usual, sans the usual scarring, the researcher knew he was onto something. He delved into the study of essential oils, documenting their effects on various conditions.

An aromatherapy massage therapist is a person who holds enhanced massage therapy training with additional schooling in aromatherapy techniques.

Aromatherapy has two ways to access the body; via the olfactory system and through absorption into the skin. The olfactory system, that is, everything related to your sense of smell and taste, is connected to the limbic system, which regulates the emotions. What you smell can influence your hormone production and stimulate your nervous system, as well as affecting your heart rate, your blood pressure, and your respiratory system.

In aromatherapy, oils are applied to the skin, penetrating deep down into the muscles, relaxing or stimulating them, depending on the specific essential oil that is used.

Essential oils are often utilized in tandem with a variety of massage techniques, most notably Swedish massage, but also as part of lymphatic, neuromuscular, or reflexology massage therapies. Each essential oil contains unique healing properties, which can be applied strategically by a trained therapist to treat specific issues.

## Benefits

The oils used are completely natural and are applied to the outside of the body. Aromatherapy massage can be applied to infants and the elderly, as well as virtually everyone in between. A gentle rub down with some highly diluted lavender lotion may help a baby sleep at night. Rosemary or peppermint may invigorate an elderly person.

Essential oils encourage the body's natural healing process to be more efficient. The oils warm the skin and bring the blood to the surface, thus increasing circulation. With the increase in circulation, toxins begin to move out of the body. As the oils absorb through the skin, they move into the blood stream and make their way to the deepest parts of the body.

Aromatherapy massage has been known to help insomniacs sleep better. It can minimize recurring headaches, relieve the symptoms of PMS, and alleviate chronic back pain. It can be a great ally in fighting depression and anxiety. Anyone with circulatory, breathing, nerve, or immune system problems can benefit from strategic aromatherapy massage.

## Contraindications

Avoid aromatherapy massage if you have a skin rash or an open wound, because the oils may aggravate your condition. As with all massage, avoid it following surgery, if you have problems with blood clots, if you have a fever or a cold, or if you have recently received chemotherapy or radiation treatments. Pregnant women can benefit from aromatherapy massage, but be careful to employ only therapists who are specifically trained in pregnancy massage.

## How it Works

The Egyptians distilled plants in order to make essential oils and used them in rituals for the dead, as medicines, and as perfume. Part of the Roman bath consisted of indulging in fragrant and healing oils.

Aromatherapy has been employed as a healing modality for centuries, so pairing it with massage is only natural. French biochemist, Marguerite Maury, first paired aromatherapy with massage techniques in the early 1900s, and thus aromatherapy massage was born.

## How it Works

The use of essential oils differentiates aromatherapy massage from other types of massage, but there is also another difference. The focus is on utilizing the oils effectively, so the specific massage is secondary in importance. Swedish massage techniques are employed with a very light touch, as it is more important to introduce the essential oils to the skin and pull the blood up to the skin's surface to facilitate absorption than it is to work kinks and lumps out of muscles.

Each oil has its own therapeutic qualities. The aromatherapist must be well versed in healing with essential oils and must know which oils to combine in order to most effectively serve the client. At the same time, the oil must smell good. Often, a therapist will blend two or three different oils and suspend them in a carrier oil.

Treatment is usually performed with the client lying naked on a table but covered with a cloth. If this is uncomfortable, the therapist will usually allow the client to wear underclothing or remain partially clothed. A massage session is usually scheduled for an hour. This gives the oils enough time to enter the blood stream and travel throughout the body.

In aromatherapy massage, the oils are applied all over the body. They must remain on the skin for at least six hours in order to adequately do their job. Consequently, clients should avoid heavy exercise, showering or bathing during that time. They should also sip water frequently during this time to remove toxins from the body. The effects of an aromatherapy massage may be noticed for up to 48 hours.

## Techniques

The oil is applied to the body in strokes that are long and sweeping. This helps to warm the skin and underlying tissues. Following a warm-up, the therapist will usually proceed with kneading and other Swedish massage techniques performed much lighter and more gently than actual Swedish massage. The focus is on blending the aroma and the absorbed therapeutic essences with touch.

Here is a brief summary of essential oils that have been used effectively to treat specific conditions.

**Aches and Pains** – Clove, rosemary and cypress oils help increase circulation and aid in muscle recovery and cell regeneration. These oils can help recovery after you've over-exerted yourself. In addition to these oils, clary sage can relieve menstrual pain.

**Inflammation and Insomnia** – Oregano, lavender, German chamomile and patchouli are good for inflammations. These oils reduce the inflammation and ease pain. Adding lavender can also help insomnia as it relaxes the body and mind. It may also stimulate pleasant dreams.

**Circulation Issues** – Mint contains a high amount of menthol, which will increase circulation by stimulating the area of the brain that releases noradrenalin. This hormone also helps to increase the attention span. Rosemary is another circulation stimulant.

**Anxiety and Depression** – Lavender, chamomile, vetiver, citrus, and Clary sage help to decrease anxiety and irritability while promoting a feeling of inner peace. Citrusy scents like lemon, orange, and lime as well as geranium, lemon grass, and verbena can help reduce depression.

## Other Useful Oils

- Eucalyptus oil helps with nasal congestion. It clears the sinuses and allows you to breathe more easily.

- Frankincense oil helps if you are plagued with strong emotions you cannot control; it also helps to minimize nightmares.

- Geranium oil can moderate the symptoms of menopause and PMS; it is sometimes used to treat painful periods.

- Lavender Oil helps one relax.

- Mint will give you extra stamina.

- Sandalwood is a digestive aid and also eases dry skin.

- Tea Tree Oil is anti-fungal, germicidal and antibacterial; it can clear up skin infections and inflammation issues.

## Equipment

The massage recipient lies on a table or any flat surface. Linen sheets can be used to drape the participant during the massage. The practitioner of aromatherapy massage will use an array of essential oils along with carrier oils in the course of treatment.

## What To Expect

Before you subject yourself to aromatherapy massage you will want to satisfy yourself that the therapist is using oils they call "aromatherapy grade" or "clinical grade." You want to avoid fragrance grade or "redistilled" synthetic oils. Redistilled oils are FDA approved as food grade, are okayed for internal ingestion, but lack many of the effective ingredients important to aromatherapy. Most professional practitioners are well aware of this distinction and will be happy to provide information regarding the quality of the oils they use.

Notify your therapist if you will be in the sun for a prolonged time following therapy, as certain essential oils can increase your skin's sun sensitivity. You don't want to risk a painful burn after your nice restorative massage!

To get the most out of your aromatherapy session, I advise you to prepare your mind, body, and emotions beforehand by feeding them positive sensory experiences. Drink herbal tea or a smoothie to set the detoxification process into motion. If you can, treat yourself to a long, leisurely walk out in nature before going in to your therapy session. Listen to soothing music or engage in painting, drawing, sculpture, or other forms of hand-on creative work. You may find it particularly useful to soak in a warm bath or a hot tub before an aromatherapy massage. This serves to relax both mind and muscles, readying them to receive maximum benefit from the treatment to follow.

You will be required to remove your clothing and allow your body to be tastefully covered with draping cloths, since the massage consists of applying essential oils directly onto the skin. Your therapist will often shield your skin from possible irritation by the essential oils by first applying a carrier oil to the area to be treated. The most common carrier oils are olive, coconut, or almond oil.

Following a massage treatment, your skin may feel slightly greasy, but avoid the urge to shower for at least six hours. Do not drink alcohol during this time, as it can increase the effects of the massage beyond a comfortable level.

An aromatherapy massage may relax you so much you may want to fall asleep, so be careful if you plan to drive home.

Contact dermatitis is a possible side effect from the use of aromatherapy. Your practitioner will test first for allergic symptoms before spreading the oil over the body. Gas and increased bowel activity may appear, an indication that toxins are exiting the body. You also might find increased mucus in the nose, throat and chest, for the same reason.

# Chapter 13: Pregnancy Massage

The first texts describing massage during pregnancy come from India and Greece. These describe a woman being massaged throughout pregnancy, during labor, and following delivery to facilitate healing. Ayurvedic medicine from India has always supported massage for pregnant women and there are ancient scrolls describing methods that go back more than a thousand years. In the cold north, there are writings of Eskimos describing how a woman was massaged during labor. Massage has been utilized in Greece for women during childbirth from ancient days.

## Benefits

Massage during pregnancy is a controversial topic. Some experts advise to avoid massage during the first trimester, citing an increased risk of miscarriage during this time, but there is no conclusive evidence to support this. Others hold that massage can be beneficial to a pregnant woman at any time during the pregnancy, because it relaxes the muscles and pregnant women can use all the relaxation they can get. One major benefit of massage is the resolution of tenderness due to muscle stress, something pregnant women experience increasingly over nine months.

Carrying a baby shifts a woman's balance point, requiring her to adjust both her posture and her gait. These changes call into play muscles that are not normally used. The additional weight of carrying a baby can add stress to muscles and joints unaccustomed to bearing such loads. In addition, pregnancy can cause swelling in hands, feet, legs, and associated joints.

Massage can alleviate some of these discomforts, but it must be accomplished with care to avoid damaging both mother and baby. When a woman is pregnant, her blood thickens to minimize loss of blood during delivery, but this also leaves her vulnerable to blood clot development. Consequently, therapists will avoid deep tissue massage that could dislodge these clots.

Pregnancy massage is adapted to the skeletal and muscular adjustments in the mother's body and is designed to address irritated nerves and improve the circulation of both mother and baby.

Pregnancy massage relaxes muscles and relieves minor aches and pains. It minimizes edema, or swelling, by releasing fluids that collect in the body due to reduced circulation. Massage can treat sciatica, or nerve pain due to impingement and inflammation. It can reduce the headaches that come with pregnancy and can improve sleep throughout. Pregnancy massage releases beneficial hormones, including norepinephrine, and serotonin, both of which help to balance stress and stabilize mood. Massage can reduce the presence of cortisol, the stress hormone, and helps to keep anxiety and depression at bay. Light massage can also assist during labor

## Contraindications

You should not undergo massage therapy if you are nauseous or vomiting, or are suffering from morning sickness. You should also forego pregnancy massage if you have a high-risk pregnancy. This would include pregnancy-induced hypertension, a tendency toward preeclampsia, severe swelling, or if you have miscarried in the past or have experienced pre-term labor.

## How it Works

Even the baby can benefit from massage. The data now show that babies born to mothers who have received regular massage treatments are healthier overall. The mothers benefit by reduced pain perception during labor and both mother and child are helped by shorter and easier labor.

Any number of massage modalities may be used as part of pregnancy massage. The therapy differs primarily in the position in which the participant is placed. Beyond the 21st week, a pregnant woman should not lie on her back; the weight of the baby can impair circulation of some major blood vessels. Beyond this point – and even earlier if needed - pregnant women will be treated while lying on one side. Often the left side is preferred for reasons of circulation. The head will be supported with a pillow, and wedges or additional pillows can provide stability.

Massage, or more accurately in this case, strategic touch, is also helpful during the birthing process. One's partner can be trained to assist, but women may be helped most by therapy administered via a trained midwife or doula.

## Techniques

Pregnancy massage refers to any type of massage administered to a pregnant woman. As such, a variety of modalities are employed. Deep pressure massage should definitely be avoided, but Shiatsu tapping can be useful, when administered carefully and in the right places. Strong pressure should never be applied to the legs because it could dislodge a clot. Light wide strokes should be used on the legs. Massage on the abdomen should be avoided as well.

Many massage therapists avoid the area between the ankle and the heel, because this spot corresponds to the uterus and the ovaries. Some reflexologists hold that excessive pressure on this area may result in premature labor, but other professionals, trained in the details of pregnancy and massage therapy, confidently work the ankle area throughout the entire pregnancy to provide the mother much needed energy and to stimulate blood circulation to the growing infant.

Shiatsu and acupressure massage may be useful in inducing labor, but these modalities require considerable skill to be effective. They may also require treatments over an extended period of time before results occur.

Abdominal breathing has great benefits for a pregnant woman. It can work in tandem with massage to aid in muscle relaxation and to stimulate circulation. Controlled breathing can reduce pain both throughout the pregnancy and during labor.

Throughout labor, massage in the form of light stroking can help remove lactic acid buildup from muscles. This therapy is performed when the woman is resting between contractions. Stroking also stimulates nerves to reduce the perception of pain.

# Chapter 14: Myofascial Massage

Myofascial Massage is a newer therapy that developed in the United States. It treats the body's fascia. Fascia is a thin, protective membrane-like substance that extends throughout every muscle, every nerve, every bone, artery, vein and organ in the body. Think of it as one continuous sweater over the inside of the body or imagine a big spider web that stretches continuously in and out of every physical system.

The fascia surrounds everything and holds together all the components of the body. Certain events – such as trauma or inflammation – can cause the fascia, which is normally stretchy and pliable, to become tight and hard. Surgery may cause the fascia to harden, especially if scar tissue forms. When portions of the fascia are hardened, this is considered a restriction. These restrictions prevent lymphatic fluids from passing freely throughout the body to eliminate toxins.

Myofascial massage is also termed skin rolling or myofascial release. Treatment is a mixture of kneading, light stretching, and other massage techniques. The therapist gently applies pressure to the myofascial tissues in order to remove pain and restrictions.

One good example is frozen shoulder. When you have a frozen shoulder, your range of motion is very limited. You may not be able to reach up, down or very far backwards. Myofascial massage helps to increase the range of motion. The slow and consistent application of pressure allows the fascia to stretch and elongate, easing restrictions. Myofascial restrictions are seldom detectable by CAT scans, X-rays or other diagnostic protocols, but they exist all the same and myofascial massage can ease them.

## Benefits

Myofascial massage does ease pain and increases range of motion. It also corrects imbalances in muscles. The following are just a few conditions that myofascial massage can improve.

Carpal Tunnel – This condition affects the hands and compresses the nerves, making it very painful to pick up anything or to type. Myofascial massage can increase pliability in the area.

Cervical and Lumbar issues – The shoulders and back can grow stiff because of lifting heavy objects or repetitive movements. Myofascial massage can remove the pain and facilitate spinal flexibility.

Headaches and Migraines – The fascia extends to the head and throughout the brain. Headaches may be caused by many things, including trauma to the neck or head, stress, and poor posture. The fascia becomes tight before a headache begins. Massage releases the tightness and allows posture to improve and neck alignment to return to normal.

During a woman's menstrual cycle, it is possible for the fascia to become tight due to stomach bloating and the additional pressure it engenders. Myofascial massage can make the resulting cramps disappear.

Chronic Fatigue and Fibromyalgia – Both of these conditions can cause a great deal of pain, which often stems from restrictions in the fascia. Massage treatment can increase the pliability of the fascia and stop most of the pain with an added benefit of enhancing healthy sleep.

Spine Issues – A displaced or bulging disc in the back is a major cause of pain. Misalignment can cause deterioration that massage can arrest. At least it can stop further disc herniation and remove some of the pain.

Plantar Fasciitis – This condition applies to the arch of the foot, where a band of tissue wraps around it. This tissue can become inflamed and misalign the bones in the foot. Massage relieves the tightness and resolves much of the foot discomfort.

Sciatica – This condition arises when the sciatic nerve, which runs down the back, buttocks and upper leg, receives undue pressure from swollen muscles. It can create painful muscle spasms that make it difficult to sit or stand. Massage can decrease these spasms and release the compression that is irritating the nerve.

Scoliosis – Scoliosis is an unhealthy curvature of the spine. While massage cannot cure this condition, it can make it more manageable by restoring alignment and pliability to the fascia.

TMJ Syndrome – Myofascial massage has been found to relieve some of the symptoms of TMJ.

Myofascial massage can also strengthen the immune system, it can help a sluggish lymphatic system to flow and can increase the circulation of all fluids through the body.

## How it Works

Andrew Taylor Still, known as the father of osteopathy, published *Myofascial Pain & Dysfunction: The Trigger Point Manual* in 1976. The term "myofascial release" was coined by Robert Ward, an osteopath who was familiar with physical therapy. Ward worked with a physical therapist named John Barnes and explored the technique called Rolfing. Ward and Barnes are considered the founders of myofascial release.

## Description

Myofascial massage is accomplished without the aid of oils or creams. It takes 45 minutes to one hour to complete a massage. The participant lies face down on a table with the back uncovered. A therapist, using the pads of the thumb and fingers, picks up a roll of skin next to the spine. He will hold it for a few seconds and then slowly begin to roll it up the spine, lifting it away from the underlying tissue. If performed correctly, the therapist will move a continuous roll of skin from the bottom of the body to its top. As the roll progresses, a therapist will look for signs of pain. Whenever he reaches a spot that is painful, he will employ other massage methods to relax the fascia and remove any restrictions that are generating the pain.

## Techniques

One of the simplest procedures used in this type of massage is the **strain-counterstrain** technique. The therapist finds a position in which participants are completely comfortable and lets them lie there for a while. Often, this will release restrictions in the fascia without additional manipulation.

**Kneading** and **trigger point** work are also part of Myofascial massage. These strategies loosen muscles and fascial tissue so that the fascia can revert to its normal shape. Gentle pressure is held for about two minutes on severe restrictions before being released. The pressure is gentle; nothing like the hard pressure used in trigger point massage.

Self myofascial massage is possible; ideally, you will be trained in these techniques by a qualified therapist. Often, therapists utilize a variety of foam rollers as part of their therapy, but these tools are easily replicated for home use.

## How It Works

The participant lies on a foam roll to create pressure, then rolls the body along it to massage the fascia and release restrictions. This can be performed while lying on the back, on the side, on the stomach or on other areas of concern. The participant can roll both up and down and from side to side.

Myofascial release can also be performed using nothing but the hands. This gives therapists the advantage of being able to feel blockages in the fascia and address them as they work.

## Equipment

The participant lies on a foam mat or a therapy table. Foam cylinders used as tools work well on large muscle groups. They can be used to massage the hamstrings, quads, and the back. Rollers are either dense or soft and also come in the form of high density PVC pipe that has a hard core. Grid rollers and small rollers can be used on your quadriceps. There is even a roller with tiny bumps called a rumble roller.

However, rollers aren't absolutely required; you can use balls to the same end. Golf balls work well on the feet while tennis balls help shoulders, gluts and back. A Lacrosse ball is good for quads and hamstrings as well as pectoral muscles and the front area of the hip. A medicine ball works well on the shoulders and upper back.

## Benefits

Myofascial massage can stop pain in its tracks. It can also be used as a preventative modality to keep the fascia pliable. This form of massage can help your body recover from physical trauma, including surgery, and can help with chronic severe pain. It is also helpful in treating grief, anxiety, and depression.

# Chapter 15: Reflexology Massage

The goal of reflexology massage is to release any blockages to the flow of energy. This is accomplished by applying pressure to reflex points. These points – located in the feet, hands, and ears – correlate to other areas of the body. It is thought that the body repairs itself once a blockage or "restriction" is released.

When pressure is applied, it relays signals by way of the nervous system to related areas of the body, encouraging those areas to relax and allow energy to flow freely to the area. For example, there is a spot on the feet that, when pressure is applied, will relieve a headache. Charts for the hands, feet, and ears have been developed over the centuries so that the related parts of the body and their reflex points are easily identified.

## Benefits

Reflexology massage is said to facilitate the flow of healing energy throughout the body. The benefits are many and include reducing headaches and migraines, lowering blood pressure, easing PMS and menopause symptoms in women, stopping the swelling in feet and legs, aiding in the healing of injuries, stopping the pain of plantar fasciitis, and help for the symptoms of chronic fatigue syndrome and fibromyalgia.

## Contraindications

Avoid foot reflexology if you have had a foot fracture; signals to other parts of the body may be impeded in this case. Individuals with varicose veins or a tendency to develop blood clots should avoid reflexology massage as it may cause clots to dislodge. Anyone with active gout or open foot wounds should avoid foot reflexology, but the technique can still be performed on hands and ears.

## How it Works

While reports of treatments similar to reflexology can be traced back to ancient Egypt and China, the profession – as we now know it – did not come into being until the late 19th Century.

A neurologist from England in the 1890s named Sir Henry Head researched how pressure points on one part of the body can help cure another part of the body. In the early 1900s, William Fitzgerald, an American ear, nose and throat doctor, experimented with applying pressure on one side of the body to effect areas on the other side.

In the 1930s Eunice Ingham, a physiotherapy nurse, took his idea and expanded it. She realized that the hands and feet were very sensitive and ultimately drew up the first reflexology charts. In 1968, her nephew, Dwight Byers, founded the National Institute of Reflexology.

Theories abound, but nobody really knows how reflexology helps a body to heal. What we have, however, are thousands of pieces of anecdotal evidence that support its effectiveness.

## Description

In reflexology massage, there is no need to remove any clothing except shoes and socks. The therapist or practitioner only works with the feet, the hands, the face, and/or the ears, depending on the needs of the individual client. The client is usually treated in a seated position, although some therapists have individuals lie down. Usually there are no oils used, but sometimes lotion is applied, especially if the feet are badly calloused. A massage lasts anywhere from 45 to 60 minutes. The therapist will begin at the toes and work up the foot to the heel. If the hands are treated, therapy will begin with the fingers and work toward the wrist. Ear treatment is performed from the top down to the earlobe.

When easing the pain of migraines is the goal, the toes and/or fingers are the focus. In the case of migraines, light pressure will be applied to the fingers or toes. When he was a child, my brother suffered from sudden, excruciating migraines. Quite by accident, he discovered that if he applied pressure to the web between his thumb and index finger, the headache would go away. In this way, he used reflexology principles to treat himself without knowing it as such.

## Techniques

The reflexology therapist employs several unique techniques during a treatment session:

**Thumb Walking** is the most common technique used in order to find and treat congestion or restrictions. The thumb is bent and straightened repeatedly which moves or "walks" it across the client's hand or foot. A trained therapist can tell from tension under the pad of the thumb whether any congestion exists, and provide resolution.

**Twist and Wring** is another common technique designed to remove restrictions. The therapist uses both hands with the fingers on top of the foot and thumbs on the bottom. The hands are then slowly twisted or wrung away from one another to create tension on the sole of the foot.

**Rotation** consists of holding a toe or finger at its base and moving the entire digit in a circular motion to release tightness.

## Equipment

The therapist needs little more than a good set of hands to accomplish this treatment. While a trained professional is more certain to identify and treat your ailments, it is possible to treat yourself. Your therapist can point out key spots for you to treat between sessions and can check to ensure you are applying the correct pressure in the appropriate location.

If you choose to treat yourself independently, you will need reflexology charts for the hands, feet, and ears to indicate where to apply pressure.

A professional will usually treat you while you are seated in a chair. Some reflexologists use a foam foot roller on the bottom of the foot, but this is not mandatory.

## Contraindications

There are only a few people for which reflexology massage is *not* recommended. You should forego treatment opportunities if you have any of the following conditions:

- Deep vein thrombosis

- A risky pregnancy

- The first two weeks following a stroke

- A fever

There are possible side effects to reflexology massage, but none of them are terrible. You might feel cold for a while or light headed right after a massage. This is largely due to increased oxygen to areas that are not used to it. The massage may also relax you enough to make you feel sleepy.

Even if you don't feel thirsty after a massage, you should drink plenty of water in order to flush the out the toxins that were released by the therapy. Toxins may also be flushed out in the form of mucus from the nose or bowels and you may experience a bit of a rash or pimples, but these should subside shortly.

# Chapter 16: Lymphatic Massage

Lymphatic massage first was developed in France by a husband and wife team from Denmark, Emil Vodder, PhD and his wife, Estrid, a naturopath. They first began to develop lymphatic treatments during the 1930s in France.

Dr. Vodder, born in Copenhagen, was stricken with malaria while he was in medical school. After recovering from his illness, he was unable to continue his education in medicine, receiving instead a PhD in Historical Art.

This might seem to preclude him from inventing a form of therapeutic massage, but his interest in historical art contributed to its development. The couple had moved to the French Riviera where Emil was devoting himself to researching the extant literature on what were then called the lymph organs (today's lymph nodes). One day, Emil discovered some ancient copper engravings by an anatomist named Sappey. These engravings showed a technique for hand pumping and light massage in circular movements over the skin.

Dr. Vodder researched further. Ultimately, the husband and wife team began to develop techniques for what we know as lymphatic massage. Emil was personally invested in the treatment because he was frequently plagued by serious sinus infections and colds.

In the 1960s German physician Dr. Asdonk became acquainted with Vodder's studies and extended them, creating a list of common indications. In 1966, Gunter Wittlinger became acquainted with Dr. Vodder's work; he opened the first Vodder school in 1967. This new method of massage came to North America in 1972 and a Vodder school was opened in 1993.

While the blood, or circulatory system has a pump called the heart that moves blood around the body; the lymph system has to depend on gravity. This system is further aided by lymph nodes found in the body, with major nodes situated in the neck, underarms and the groin area. These nodes assist in the filtering of waste products. Lymph vessels are found right under the skin, so only gentle pressure is needed in this form of massage.

Lymphatic massage is primarily used to treat lymphedema, an accumulation of lymph fluids due to a poorly performing lymph system or a compromised lymph system, such as when a lymph node must be removed in the treatment of cancer. In the latter case, when cancerous tissue is removed, the nearby lymph nodes are often taken out as well.

## Benefits

There is some controversy about lymphatic massage. Some doctors say you don't need it unless a lymph node has been removed, but others believe it can benefit almost everyone. The massage has been found helpful in regaining energy after being sick or following an injury or surgery, even if lymph nodes were not affected.

When scar tissue is forming, it creates a little swelling in the process. Lymphatic massage cannot prevent scarring, but can render the scar thinner and less noticeable. It can help individuals who have swelling in their arms, hands, legs and feet. People who struggle with acne can benefit from the massage, as it removes inflammations and can reduce the swelling of pimples.

Individuals with chronic fatigue or fibromyalgia may find relief through this massage modality. Pregnant women can also benefit. Often, hormone changes create edema during pregnancy, but lymphatic massage can prevent this swelling. It can also help women who have suffer from PMS and can help breast-feeding mothers by keeping their breast tissue soft and supple.

## How it Works

To understand what Lymphatic massage does, you must understand a little bit about the body's lymph system. This system runs through the body and washing wastes and toxins picked up in lymph fluid that lies in the space between cells. You can think of it as a giant filtering tree with small roots near the skin's surface that branch into larger vessels flowing into the blood system. Lymph fluid is whitish to clear and it is important that it doesn't get hung up anywhere and start to collect. If it does, it causes swelling, immune issues and can encourage the growth of viruses and bacteria, leading to an all-out physical infection.

Congestion can lead to colds, the flu, and increase fatigue. When lymph fluid is allowed to flow freely, the body remains healthy and our immune system works effectively to ward off infection. Lymphatic massage can flush the lymphatic system, enabling it to work to the best of its ability, as it aids in the clearing of wastes and toxins from the system.

## Description

Lymphatic Massage is very gentle. Often, it employs the use of just the fingers and the palms. There is no heavy pressure in this modality, just light, constant, rhythmic movement across the surface of the skin. A massage session will last from 45 to 60 minutes. It usually focuses on lymph node areas The massage is not painful yet it is stimulating and those who have had a node removed will need this stimulation more frequently than anyone who has all lymph nodes intact

The massage begins at the neck and goes toward the ears, to the temple, the forehead, and back to the neck. A whole body massage will continue by massaging the arms, from the hands up to underarm. Legs are massaged beginning with the feet and moving on up toward the groin area.

## Techniques

There are four main techniques used during the massage. Keep in mind that with lymphatic massage, the movement is always toward the heart.

**Stationary Circles** – The fingers work in continuous spirals over the skin of the neck and face. This motion directs fluids toward the location of the lymph nodes and, ultimately, the heart.

**Pumping** – The palms are placed flat on the skin and moved in oval strokes with the aid of thumbs and fingers. This helps to stimulate the flow of fluids.

**Rotary** – With this technique, the massage goes in cylindrical movements with the palms flat on the body. The wrists are used to increase and decrease light pressure.

**Scoop Strokes** – The therapist makes a scoop shape with the hand, extending the fingers and bending the hand. The hands grab a bit of the skin with a brief twisting stroke before it is released.

The pressure should never be harsh. Hands should slide on the skin but the hands should never really sense anything under the skin. If they do, the therapist is pressing too hard. Pushing too hard can collapse the lymph organ, preventing fluids from being released.

The rhythm behind all of these techniques is constant, allowing fluid to be sucked out of the lymph organs and into the blood, to be flushed out of the body.

## Contraindications

Avoid lymphatic massage if you have a cold, the flu or another infection, because this therapy can spread your illness to other parts of the body. If you have extreme swelling following surgery, do not see a massage therapist for help. Instead, speak immediately to your doctor.

Individuals with congestive heart failure should avoid this massage because large amounts of fluids collect in this condition, more than the massage can safely evacuate. If you currently have cancer or any malignant or metastatic condition, you should wait until the area has been removed or completely healed before pursuing lymphatic treatment.

There are few side effects to this type of massage because it is so gentle. In extreme cases, nausea, vomiting, or bruising of the skin may occur. Diabetics may need to take in nourishment during treatment and immediately following it to avoid sugar imbalances. If you are a diabetic, this massage may impact your sugar levels for several hours following a massage.

# Chapter 17: How To Select A Therapist

Now that you've explored a variety of massage techniques, you might be feeling a little overwhelmed with the multitude of possible choices. This chapter will help you navigate the various options and choose which will best serve your needs.

Each body is different; what helps you may be completely irrelevant to someone else. At the same time, each therapist is a unique individual with a one-of-a-kind mix of personality, skills, training, and experience. Because of this double uniqueness, you may need to try out several therapists and pursue several different types of massage therapy before you find a person with the skill sets, the personality and the right sensitivities to help you best.

This chapter is designed to help you pull together the traits of the various forms of massage so that you can more easily discern which forms of massage will do you the most good. Keep in mind that as your life progresses, your physical, mental, and emotional needs will change; consequently, your massage needs may shift, requiring adjustments in your treatment. I recommend you re-evaluate your massage needs periodically and whenever significant changes occur in your life.

At the end of the chapter, I will conclude by outlining some basic principles to use when selecting a therapist. I have noted things to look for and dangers to avoid, in order to establish the best ongoing relationship possible and to maximize your results.

## Self-Massage

With a plethora of massage training videos added daily to the internet, it raises the question, why can't I just treat myself? You may be looking to save money, or perhaps you just prefer the do-it-yourself approach. At any rate, this is a question worth looking into.

The advantage of self-massage is that you can sometimes feel your body responding to your treatment. This is especially helpful in trigger point therapy, where you definitely know when you've located a trigger point – it hurts! You can also feel the trigger point start to dissolve. Of course, a professional is trained to locate trigger points by touch and can feel them resolve, but self-massage can be highly beneficial, and it can save you a lot of money.

There are other advantages to self-massage. By doing so, you take the responsibility for your health into your own hands, quite literally! Ownership of your health is always a good thing. Self-massage also serves as a form of self-soothing and self-nurturing. If you are learning to take care of yourself, following years of neglect or self-hate, this practice can build positive qualities into your life. It can help you feel good about the kind of person you are. It can also build your confidence in your capability to take care of yourself.

## Professional Massage Therapists

In most cases, with massage therapy you get what you pay for. Self-taught massage therapists, largely of the whole-body massage type, can do much good, just as a shoulder massage from a friend can help relax you when tense or tired. I have a relative who has taught herself a mixture of Swedish, Shiatsu, trigger point massage and reflexology. Whenever I visit her, I am treated to a wonderfully relaxing massage that often resolves my current aches and pains.

In America, our rugged individualism easily leads to a touch-free existence. Unless you have been blessed with a touchy-feely family of origin, you may have grown up starved for physical touch, yet unaware and/or unable to bridge the physical gap between yourself and others. A professional massage therapist can bridge the gap, teaching your body to thrive under nurturing touch and helping you become comfortable in social settings that require it.

A professionally trained massage therapist will have a depth and breadth of knowledge that is missing in most self-trained practitioners. To achieve certification, a therapist receives training in human physiology, learning the normal skeletal structure, musculature, and nervous system, as well as the location and function of the internal organs. A therapist is also trained in a wide variety of massage techniques, learning their correct applications and knowing when – and more importantly, when not – to employ them for the greater good.

As part of certification training, a therapist learns how touch can harm as well as heal. This is knowledge your Aunt Sally may have not acquired in the course of her self-training. There are certain types of touch that can injure a person, no matter which massage modality is chosen. Professionals will be quite knowledgeable, not only regarding what to do, but also in what to avoid.

The more specialized or complex your needs, the more important it is to employ the services of a trained professional. You want to be confident you are in the hands of someone who knows the interplay of your symptoms and the side effects of each possible treatment.

## There Is Another Way

Personally, I prefer a combination of professional therapy and professionally directed self-massage. I rely on my massage therapist to help me learn ways I can treat myself in between sessions. This gives me the best of both worlds.

My own bodywork is overseen by a professional who gives me feedback to ensure that what I do is performed correctly. I have a wonderful therapist who is willing to take the time to help me grow in my understanding of my body; he is professional, yet patiently answers my questions and gives generously of his knowledge.

## Massage Therapies, Summarized

Massage therapies fall into one of two general categories: Whole-body relaxation massage and therapies that address specific needs. If you just need to de-stress or relax your whole body, Swedish massage, a chair massage, or hot stone therapy will serve you well.

If you are going in for your first massage, choose one of the above. It will introduce you to the basic techniques common to all forms of massage therapy and you will come away feeling refreshed and reinvigorated. Later, if you wish, you can always move on to other forms of massage.

## Address Specific Needs With The Right Tools

Just as you would never use a hammer to affix a screw, you will want to select a massage "tool" that best fits your needs. While most massage therapies are like a Swiss army knife in that they have a positive influence on multiple conditions, a few modalities are highly specialized and designed to treat specific diagnoses. Here is a summary of the different massage therapies covered in this book, along with some reported uses and benefits:

- Aromatherapy Massage – Headache, stress, PMS, digestion, as well as facilitation of other massage modalities

- Deep Tissue Massage – Chronic deep muscle pain, stiff muscles, high blood pressure, scar tissue, range of motion

- Erotic Massage – Stress, premature ejaculation, tension

- Lymphatic Massage – Lymph fluid drainage (lymphedema), sinus infections, inflammation, scarring, edema (swelling)

- Myofascial Massage – fibromyalgia, migraines, range of motion, PMS

- Neuromuscular Massage – Blood circulation, posture

- Pregnancy Massage – Pregnancy, labor, post-delivery recovery

- Reflexology Massage – All areas of the body, most notably organ stimulation, PMS, fibromyalgia, headaches

- Shiatsu Massage – Chi flow, making muscles limber, fibromyalgia, depression, anxiety, skin problems, digestion

- Sports Massage – The highly active body, repetitive motion injuries, soft tissue injuries, swelling

- Swedish Massage – Relaxation, circulation, detoxification

- Tantric Massage – spinning (balancing) the chakras, body awareness, sexual performance

- Thai Massage – Flexibility, range of motion, circulation, energy

- Trigger Point Massage – pain reduction, muscle strength, TMJ, muscle spasms

## Choose Wisely

Finding a good massage therapist can be challenging, but it need not be stressful. Here are a few tips to ensure you find a massage therapist that is right for you.

1. Know what you want. It's important that you start out with a clear idea of what you want to see accomplished. While your needs will change over time, go with what you need now. This will help you choose a therapist who has the skills that you need.

2. What massage types from the list above best match what you need in a massage? Keep in mind that many massage therapists are skilled in multiple massage modalities. You might want write down the necessary massage skills in a must-have list. While you're at it, make a separate wish list for things you would like, but that aren't essential. You will be looking for a therapist with all the skills on your "must have" list, and then anything you find on your wish list will be an added bonus.

3. Think about what massage techniques you are comfortable with and also specify anything that you want to rule out. You will need to communicate this with your therapist. Remember, while your therapist is very sensitive to your body's cues, he or she cannot read your mind; it's best to be as up-front as possible from the start.

   If you're new to massage, let a potential therapist know, but at the same time communicate your level of willingness to try new things. There's nothing wrong about being cautious when it comes to the unknown; we can't all be like Indiana Jones. However you need the assurance that any therapist you employ is willing to work at your pace and prepare you carefully for what you will experience.

   If, at any time, you get the feeling that a potential therapist will push you beyond what you are ready for, you may want to seek out someone else.

Massage is supposed to be a positive experience, not a harrowing contest of wills.

4.  Ask for referrals from friends and acquaintances. Bear in mind that their preferences may not be yours. Still, a positive referral from someone you trust can set you on the right track to finding the therapist you are looking for.

    If you have a chiropractor or a physician you trust, ask for a referral; they may know just the person you are looking for.

5.  Interview prospective massage therapists – at least their office staff – initially by phone. The office should be willing to give you answers to basic questions such as:

    - Do their office hours work for your schedule?

    - What is the cost?

    - Is tipping recommended?

    - Will they accept your medical insurance, or

    - Do they provide a sliding scale fee for those without insurance?

6.  Note that "bodywork" is another name for reputable massage therapists, whereas the phrase "happy endings" implies the provision of sexual services, which are largely illegal.

7.  Schedule an interview with a therapist. At this interview, don't hesitate to ask the following questions – any professional therapist will have no problem answering them:

    - Are you licensed to practice in this state? A credentialed massage therapist will often have the abbreviations, CMT (Certified Massage Therapist) or LMT (Licensed Massage Therapist) following his or her name. This is an indication that the therapist is indeed cleared to practice massage therapy in your state.

    - If you are looking for a type of massage that is highly specialized, you will want to ask about certification in that specialization. For example, sports therapists will have a SMT (Sports Massage Therapist) certification while neuromuscular therapists will have NMT (Neuromuscular Therapist) credentials following the indication that they are board certified.

- You may also wish to learn if the therapist is a member of any professional organizations, such as the American Massage Therapy Association (AMTA) or the Association of Bodywork Massage Professionals (ABMP). This is not essential, but gives added credibility to a therapist.

- What oils do you use as part of a massage? This is especially important if you have any product allergies.

- What is your disinfection protocol? Most therapists will wipe down tables, etc. with a disinfectant before each client. If they don't, run for the hills.

- What is your draping practice? You want to be confident that your therapist is committed to respect your modesty and ensure your comfort throughout the massage.

Discuss in detail what you are looking for in a massage. Describe any specific issues you wish to be treated for and don't hesitate to ask if the therapist has experience in treating for those issues.

If your condition is rare, don't be surprised if the therapist lacks experience in its treatment. However, before hiring a therapist, you will want the assurance that the therapist is committed to learning about your condition and researching appropriate treatment modalities. If a therapist shows no interest in tailoring massage treatment to address your concerns, you might as well move on and find someone else who *will*.

8. If you think you've found the right therapist, or if you've narrowed the field to just a couple possibilities, I recommend scheduling a short massage. This will allow you to see if you are a good fit for each other.

9. Be patient with the process. While you may be fortunate enough to discover a great therapist right away, it is often a matter of trial and error to find the right match for your particular needs. The more specific or specialized your massage needs, the more challenging this process can be. On the other hand, your specific needs may help you narrow the field more easily. Whatever the case, it is important that you commit to being present throughout, consciously choosing the path to your optimal therapist.


## Communication is Key

Whenever you go in for a massage, it is important to communicate your expectations, likes, and dislikes, both before you engage a therapist, during the massage, and afterwards. While therapists are usually highly attuned to your body's needs and sensitivities, don't expect them to read your mind. If you like something, tell your therapist.  If a spot is sensitive or if a massage technique is uncomfortable, let your therapist know immediately.  You are paying good money for this, so there's no reason to endure something that is painful and may be harmful to your body.

When it comes right down to it, your therapist stands or falls based on the quality of the feedback you provide.  Communication is key.  It can make for an excellent massage or a less-than-stellar experience, so do your part to keep the lines of communication flowing.  Then, you will be well on your way to giving your mind and body what they need in order to function at peak performance levels.

# Conclusion

I hope this book was able to help you to decide what kind of massage therapies will help you the most. Remember to hydrate yourself well both before and following any therapeutic massage. Massage will loosen toxins and other waste products that water will help flush out of your body. The fastest way to remove those toxins is to drink plenty of water.

Your next step is to find a therapist or someone to practice your new skills on. Don't be afraid to try out the various different massage methods in this book. You can likely find at least one Swedish massage, sports massage, and deep tissue massage offered in your town. Before the start of a therapy session, inform your therapist of any recent injuries, any physical or emotional issues, and any chronic conditions you may want them to work on. Throughout the session, let your therapist know what helps and especially, anything that hurts. By letting them know where they need to focus their attention, your results will be dramatically increased! Let your massage be a pleasurable experience, one you will want to repeat again and again.

Finally, if you discovered at least one thing that has helped you or that you think would be beneficial to someone else, be sure to take a few seconds to easily post a quick positive review. As an author, your positive feedback is desperately needed. Your highly valuable five star reviews are like a river of golden joy flowing through a sunny forest of mighty trees and beautiful flowers! *To do your good deed in making the world a better place by helping others with your valuable insight, just leave a nice review.*

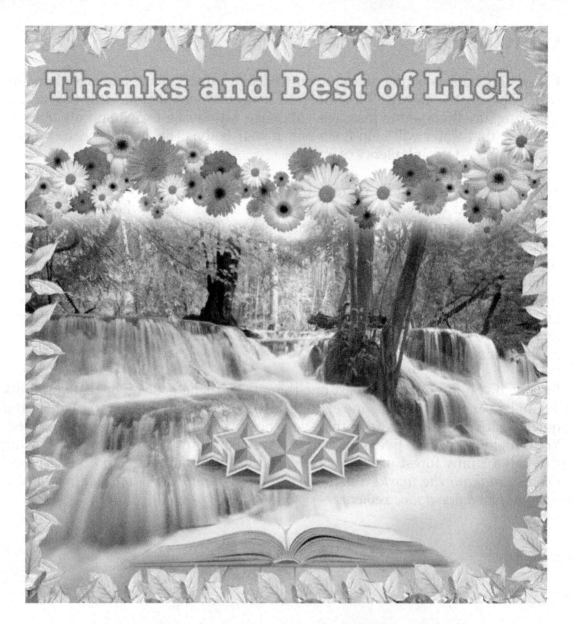

**My Other Books and Audio Books**
www.AcesEbooks.com

# Health Books

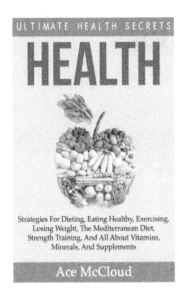

ULTIMATE HEALTH SECRETS

# HEALTH

Strategies For Dieting, Eating Healthy, Exercising, Losing Weight, The Mediterranean Diet, Strength Training, And All About Vitamins, Minerals, And Supplements

Ace McCloud

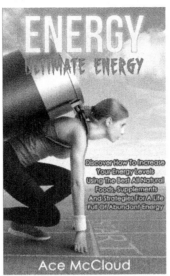

# ENERGY
## ULTIMATE ENERGY

Discover How To Increase Your Energy Levels Using The Best All Natural Foods, Supplements And Strategies For A Life Full Of Abundant Energy

Ace McCloud

# RECIPE BOOK

The Best Food Recipes That Are Delicious, Healthy, Great For Energy And Easy To Make

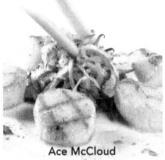

Ace McCloud

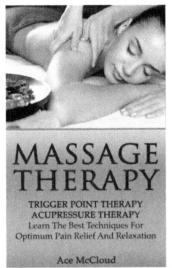

# MASSAGE THERAPY

TRIGGER POINT THERAPY
ACUPRESSURE THERAPY
Learn The Best Techniques For Optimum Pain Relief And Relaxation

Ace McCloud

# LOSE WEIGHT

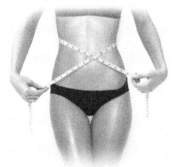

THE TOP 100 BEST WAYS TO LOSE WEIGHT QUICKLY AND HEALTHILY

Ace McCloud

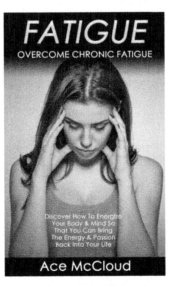

# FATIGUE
OVERCOME CHRONIC FATIGUE

Discover How To Energize Your Body & Mind So That You Can Bring The Energy & Passion Back Into Your Life

Ace McCloud

# Peak Performance Books

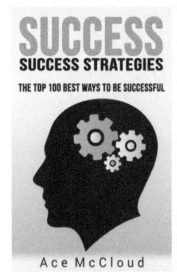

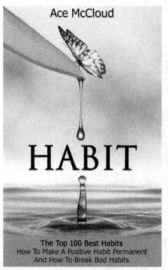

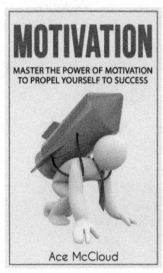

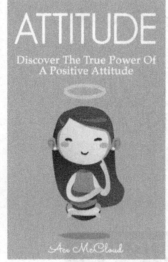

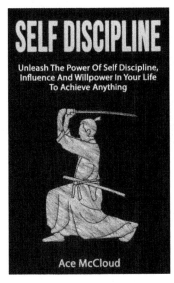

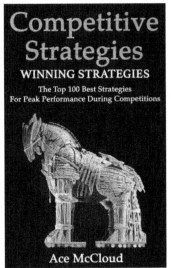

# Be sure to check out my audio books as well!

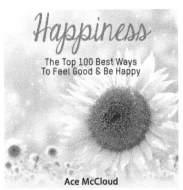

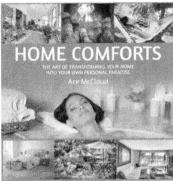

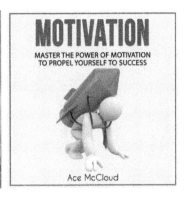

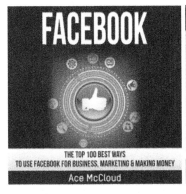

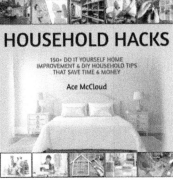

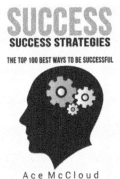

Check out my website at: **www.AcesEbooks.com** for a complete list of all of my books and high quality audio books. I enjoy bringing you the best knowledge in the world and wish you the best in using this information to make your journey through life better and more enjoyable! **Best of luck to you!**

**Be sure to check out my audio books as well**

9 781640 483026